Key Questions in Clinical Farm Animal Medicine

Volume 1

Principles of Disease Examination, Diagnosis and Management

Key Questions in Clinical Farm Animal Medicine

Volume 1
Principles of Disease Examination, Diagnosis and Management

Edited by **Tanmoy Rana**

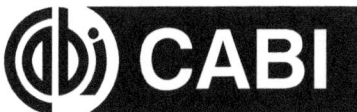

(b) CABI

CABI is a trading name of CAB International

CABI
Nosworthy Way
Wallingford
Oxfordshire OX10 8DE
UK

Tel: +44 (0)1491 832111
E-mail: info@cabi.org
Website: www.cabi.org

CABI
200 Portland Street
Boston
MA 02114
USA

Tel: +1 (617)682-9015
E-mail: cabi-nao@cabi.org

The views expressed in this publication are those of the author(s) and do not necessarily represent those of, and should not be attributed to, CAB International (CABI). Any images, figures and tables not otherwise attributed are the author(s)' own. References to internet websites (URLs) were accurate at the time of writing.

CAB International and, where different, the copyright owner shall not be liable for technical or other errors or omissions contained herein. The information is supplied without obligation and on the understanding that any person who acts upon it, or otherwise changes their position in reliance thereon, does so entirely at their own risk. Information supplied is neither intended nor implied to be a substitute for professional advice. The reader/user accepts all risks and responsibility for losses, damages, costs and other consequences resulting directly or indirectly from using this information.

CABI's Terms and Conditions, including its full disclaimer, may be found at https://www.cabi.org/terms-and-conditions/.

A catalogue record for this book is available from the British Library, London, UK.

ISBN-13: 9781800624764 (paperback)
          9781800624771 (ePDF)
          9781800624788 (ePub)

DOI: 10.1079/9781800624788.0000

Commissioning Editor: Alexandra Lainsbury
Editorial Assistant: Emma McCann
Production Editor: James Bishop

Typeset by Straive, Pondicherry, India

Contents

Contributors

Kanchan Arya, Veterinary and Animal Sciences, KVK, Gaina-Aincholi Pithoragarh, GBPUAT, Pantnagar, India.

Sonam Bhatt, Department of Veterinary Medicine, BVC, BASU, Patna, Bihar, India.

Deepika Caesar, College of Veterinary Science & Animal Husbandry, NDVSU, Rewa (MP), India.

Madhuri Dhurvey, College of Veterinary Science & Animal Husbandry, NDVSU, Jabalpur (MP), India.

Dr Ranbir S. Jatav, Department of Veterinary Medicine, College of Veterinary Science & Animal Husbandry, NDVSU, Jabalpur (MP), India.

Ranbir Singh Jatav, Hospital Superintendent, VCC, College of Veterinary Science & Animal Husbandry, NDVSU, Jabalpur (MP), India.

Anil Kumar, Department of Veterinary Medicine, BVC, BASU, Patna, Bihar, India.

Ankesh Kumar, Department of VCC, BVC, BASU, Patna, Bihar, India.

Praveen Kumar, Department of Veterinary Medicine, COVS, Lala Lajpat Rai University of Veterinary and Animal Sciences (LUVAS), Hisar, Haryana, India.

Vaishali Kumre, Department of Veterinary Medicine, College of Veterinary Science and Animal Husbandry, Jabalpur, India.

Dr Vipin Maurya, Department of Livestock Production Management, Faculty of Veterinary & Animal Sciences, IAS, RGSC – Banaras Hindu University, India.

Shashi Pradhan, Department of Veterinary Medicine, College of Veterinary Science & Animal Husbandry, NDVSU, Jabalpur (MP), India.

Dr K.S. Prasanna, Department of Veterinary Pathology, College of Veterinary & Animal Sciences, Kerala Veterinary and Animal Sciences University, Pookode, 673576 – Wayanad, Kerala, India.

Aditya Pratap, Department of Veterinary Medicine, College of Veterinary Science and Animal Husbandry, NDVSU, Jabalpur (MP), India.

Sunil Punia, Department of Veterinary Medicine, COVS, Rampura Phul, GADVASU, Ludhiana, India.

Dr Jigyasa Rana, Department of Veterinary Anatomy, Faculty of Veterinary & Animal Sciences, IAS, RGSC – Banaras Hindu University, India.

Dr Neha Rao, Veterinary Clinical Complex, College of Veterinary Science and Animal Husbandry, Kamdhenu University, Anand – 388001, India.

Akanksha Singhi, Department of Veterinary Medicine, College of Veterinary Science & Animal Husbandry, NDVSU, Jabalpur (MP), India.

Mitali Singh, Department of Veterinary Medicine, College of Veterinary Science & Animal Husbandry, NDVSU, Jabalpur (MP), India.

S. Sivaraman, Veterinary Clinical Complex, Veterinary College and Research Institute, Namakkal-1, India.

L. Sowmiya, Department of Veterinary Public Health and Epidemiology, Veterinary College and Research Institute, Orathanadu-614625, India.

D. Sumathi, Department of Veterinary Clinical Medicine, Veterinary College and Research Institute, Namakkal-1, India.

S. Yogeshpriya, Department of Veterinary Clinical Medicine, Veterinary College and Research Institute, Namakkal-1, India.

Preface

This book consists solely of multiple choice questions (MCQs), designed for anyone engaged in the study of veterinary science – in particular those aiming to take examinations such as national eligibility tests, DVM/BVSc and AH examinations – postgraduate study and junior and senior research fellowships. There are ten chapters, dealing with all aspects of farm animal medicine, compiled by a range of experienced authors, based on the most up-to-date knowledge in the field, and each including a brief introduction. The questions are analytical and comprehensive in nature and should be used alongside students' wider reading around their subject and their class-room learning.

Acknowledgements

I would like to convey my sincere gratitude to the Honourable Vice Chancellor, West Bengal University of Animal & Fishery Sciences, Kolkata, India, for providing me with the opportunity to edit this series of MCQ books. I am grateful to my all contributors who wholeheartedly helped me by providing their chapters so swiftly. I am also indebted to my colleagues for useful advice. I am thankful to all the personnel at CAB International for providing me with the opportunity to act as editor for this series. I would also like to thank my family for providing great support and the time to finalize each book.

Tanmoy Rana
Kolkata, India

Notes for users

The use of MCQs is common in formative and summative examination. MCQs are composed of one question (stem) with four possible answers, including the correct answer and several incorrect answers (distractors). One correct answer must be selected from the four possible responses to the stem. In some cases a true or false response only is requested.

1 General Concept of Diseases

Ranbir Singh Jatav, Shashi Pradhan and Mitali Singh

Introduction

A disease can be simply explained as an impairment of the normal state of an animal that interrupts, interferes with or modifies vital function. Animal disease remains a principal concern for humans because of economic losses and zoonotic disease outbreaks. Veterinary medicine deals with the study, prevention and treatment of animal diseases, not only in domesticated animals but also in wildlife. The main focus of veterinary preventive medicine is to prevent, control and eradicate disease, which is economically important for animals and agriculture.

Literature collected from ancient Greece and Rome contains references to the 'herd factor' in disease transmission. Both quarantine and slaughter were used to control outbreaks of any animal disease. Numerous attributes of animal diseases are better implied in terms of population or herd factor. Herds of livestock, rather than individual animals, are vaccinated against specific diseases.

Out of all, rinderpest (cattle plague) was one of the most important livestock diseases, which initiated the development of veterinary medicine. It was believed to spread when the Huns came to Europe in the 300s and when the Mongols invaded in the 1200s. Research indicates rinderpest was associated with the French Revolution and extensive famines in Africa. Serious outbreaks of the disease all around the world prompted the establishment of the first veterinary college (École Nationale Vétérinaire), in Lyon, France, in 1762. The foundation of World Organization for Animal Health (OIE) is also connected to rinderpest eradication.

Louis Pasteur's 'germ theory' became one of the fundamental foundations for general medicine, including veterinary medicine. After the discovery of germ theory, which states that specific microorganisms are the cause

© CAB International 2024. *Key Questions in Clinical Farm Animal Medicine Volume 1: Principles of Disease Examination, Diagnosis and Management* (ed. T. Rana) DOI: 10.1079/9781800624788.0001

of specific diseases, researchers became more concerned with domesticated animals used for food production, seeking to reduce any chances of infection spread.

Some examples of animal diseases that are quite similar to commonly occurring human diseases include chronic emphysema and hepatitis in horses, leukaemia in cattle, atherosclerosis in pigs, gastric ulcers in swine, hydrocephalus (fluid in the head) and skin allergies in many species, and urinary stones in cattle.

Infectious disease can be transmitted from a carrier (showing symptoms, or the infection may be in the subclinical stage) to a healthy individual via direct contact (through skin, droplets or via contamination through fomites). All communicable diseases are infectious but all infectious diseases are not communicable. Infectious diseases are caused due to the invasion of pathogens, including bacteria, fungi, viruses, protozoa, helminths and prions. In cases of subclinical infections, the pathogens are present inside the host body but no symptoms specific to that disease are observed. Thus, the animal may be infected but doesn't have an infectious disease. This principle is used for vaccine formulation. The infective pathogen is genetically engineered to reduce the pathogenicity so that when the host is injected, it triggers T-cell response and initiates acquired immunity against that pathogen.

Non-infectious diseases are all the disease conditions which are not caused by virulent pathogens and are not communicable. The usual causes of non-infectious diseases are hereditary or environmental factors. Many metabolic diseases are caused by an unsuitable alteration in genetics, causing disturbance in the normal physiology of the body. Excessive inbreeding (i.e. the mating of related animals) among all domesticated animal species has resulted in an inbreeding depression, causing an increase in the number of metabolic and hereditary diseases.

Examples of metabolic diseases include: overproduction or underproduction of hormones, which control specific body processes; nutritional deficiencies; poisoning from such agents as insecticides, fungicides, herbicides, fluorine and poisonous plants; and inherited deficiencies in the ability to synthesize active forms of specific enzymes, which are the proteins that control the rates of chemical reactions in the body.

Epidemiology is the branch of medicine which deals with cause and outcome of a disease in a population. In epidemiology, the diseases are segregated on the basis of certain features. The term 'sporadic' is used to describe a disease which occurs only infrequently, irregularly or occasionally in a few areas with no discernible spatial or temporal pattern. 'Endemic' describes an infection when it is present in a specific demographic area and is constantly present or maintained at a baseline level. The word 'epidemic' is derived from the Greek, where, *epi* means 'upon' or 'above' and *demos* means 'people'.

An epidemic can be explained as the rapid spread of disease to a large number of individuals within a short period of time in a given population.

A 'zoonosis' or 'zoonotic' disease is an infection which is not host-specific and can be transmitted to humans from animals (usually invertebrates) and vice versa. The most common examples of zoonosis are rabies and anthrax. Anthrax is one of the most contagious diseases of all, having no host specification, and is fatal. In epizoology, an 'epizootic' (or 'epizoötic', from the Greek *epi*, 'upon', + *zoon*, 'animal') is a disease event in a non-human animal population analogous to an epidemic in humans. High population-density is a major contributing factor to epizootics.

Disease control strategies

- **Control of infectious diseases.** Infectious diseases are caused by pathogenic organisms which divide inside the host body and cause symptoms. Control of such diseases is primarily based on either controlling the multiplication of pathogens inside the host body or providing the host body with acquired immunization. A common protocol in reducing transmission of contagious diseases is to decrease contact between carriers and healthy individuals. In the case of animals, this can be achieved by restriction of movement of infected animals and mass vaccination. Another method is biological control – for example, sterile male flies can be used to control screwworm disease. Chemicals such as pesticides, fungicides, rodenticides, disinfectants, etc., can be used as a mass prophylactic therapy. Many diseases are increased due to environmental factors like light and humidity. Diseases spread in farms occur due to improper disposal of faecal material, and housing and sanitation mismanagement. Environment plays a very important role in disease spread and animal immunity. Unhygienic milking procedures may lead to mastitis in cows and buffalo, improper cleaning of equine hooves can lead to laminitis, corn and canker. Newly-born calves and piglets may acquire the infection through their mother's milk. Another method of controlling any highly contagious disease is slaughter: killing the diseased animal after confirmation, with the aim of removing the source of infection. In the recent past, millions of poultry birds were slaughtered to prevent the transmission of disease to the human population.
- **Control of non-infectious diseases.** Control or prevention is mainly based on ruling out the cause of disease. In cases of hereditary diseases, such animals must not be used for breeding purposes. In cases of nutritional deficiencies, an appropriate balanced diet should be offered to the affected animal population. Inbreeding must be avoided to minimize the chances of mutation and new inherent disease conditions.

3

Multiple choice questions

1. **Which of the following is contraindicated while drenching a cow?**

   a. Holding the tongue

   b. Slow drenching

   c. Moderate upward lifting of the head

   d. Adding a slightly bitter medicine to the liquid

2. **For the treatment of parturient paresis, a general rule for dosing Ca is:**

   a. 0.5g/45 kg body weight

   b. 1g/45 kg body weight

   c. 1.5g/45 kg body weight

   d. 2g/45 kg body weight

3. **Which of the following is not a differential of caprine arthritis encephalitis (CAE)?**

   a. Enzootic ataxia

   b. Spinal cord abscess

   c. Cerebrospinal nematodiasis

   d. Generalized neuropathy

4. **'Harder udder' syndrome attributed to CAE virus infection is characterized by:**

   a. Firm, swollen mammary glands and agalactia at the time of parturition

   b. Firm, swollen mammary glands with oozing of straw-coloured fluid

   c. Firm, swollen udder and blood in milk at the time of parturition

   d. Swollen udder with normal milk production

5. **Coprophagia means:**

   a. Ingestion of soil

   b. Eating of faeces

    c. Eating of soap

    d. Eating nothing

6. **Which of the following tests is not used in the diagnosis of vesicular stomatitis?**

    a. ELISA

    b. CFT

    c. Virus neutralization

    d. Rose Bengal test

7. **Bovine ephemeral fever is also known as:**

    a. Three-day sickness

    b. Parturient paresis

    c. Monday-morning disease

    d. Dandy-Walker syndrome

8. **Fever with enlarged superficial lymph nodes in cross-bred calves is usually seen in:**

    a. Coccidiomycosis

    b. Piroplasmosis

    c. Theileriosis

    d. Toxoplasmosis

9. **Clinical signs such as vesicles on the lips, muzzle, dental pad, tongue, gingavae, interdigital spaces and teats, and reluctance to eat and walk, are common in cows/buffalo with:**

    a. FMD

    b. BVD

    c. IBR

    d. MDC

10. **The most rational treatment of parturient hemoglobinuria is:**

    a. Oral $Na_2 H_2 PO_4$

    b. IV $Na_2 H_2 PO_4$

c. IV $Na_2 H_2 PO_4$

d. Intravenous $Na H_2 PO_4$ and $CuSO_4$

11. **The drug of choice for the treatment of babesiosis in buffalo is:**

a. Imidocarb dipropionate

b. Ciprofloxacin

c. Oxytetracycline

d. Metronidazole

12. **Which of the following organisms gain access to the bovine udder during milking?**

a. *Staphylococcus aureus*

b. *E. Coli*

c. *Pseudomonas*

d. *Klebsiella*

13. **Hypomagnesemia is associated with all of the following except:**

a. Calves fed on a whole milk diet for several months

b. Animals grazing lush green pasture

c. Animals subjected to the stress of transport

d. Dairy cows fed on alfalfa for several weeks

14. **Which of the following is not a sign of PPR in goats?**

a. Occulo-nasal discharge

b. Swelling of knee joints

c. Diarrhoea and dehydration

d. Sore mouth with swollen lips

15. **Transboundary animal disease refers to:**

a. A fatal bacterial infection

b. An airborne infection transmitted from animals on one bank of a river to the other

    c. An infection which does not respect the territorial boundaries of different countries

    d. A viral infection in which secondary bacterial infections are very common

16. **Viruses causing pappular stomatitis, pseudocowpox and contagious ecthyma are parapox viruses that can all naturally infect:**

    a. People

    b. Cattle

    c. Goats

    d. Sheep

17. **Which of the following is not a clinico-pathologic finding of milk fever?**

    a. Hypocalcaemia

    b. Hypophosphatemia

    c. Hyperglycaemia

    d. Hypomagnesemia

18. **Which of the following is a rapid and sensitive test for the diagnosis of FMD?**

    a. ELISA

    b. CFT

    c. Serum neutralization

    d. Plaque reduction

19. **The incubation period for cowpox is:**

    a. 3–7 days

    b. 2–11 days

    c. 21–27 days

    d. 2–14 days

20. **Which is the combination of choice in theileriosis?**

    a. Buparvaquone + oxytetracycline

    b. Parvaquone + doxycycline

c. Buparvaquone + doxycycline

d. Parvaquone + oxytetracycline

21. **The most likely diagnosis for paresis immediately following calving in a Nilli Ravi buffalo is:**

a. Ketosis

b. Hypomagnesemia

c. Milk fever

d. Endotoxemia

22. **Which of the following is not a significant predisposing factor for ketosis?**

a. Retained fetal membranes

b. Metritis

c. Fatty liver

d. Hyperglycaemia

23. **Concerning nutritional muscular dystrophy, which statement is least accurate?**

a. The synonym for nutritional muscular degenerative dystrophy is white muscle disease

b. It is a non-inflammatory disease of skeletal and cardiac muscle

c. It is an inflammatory degenerative disease of skeletal and cardiac muscle

d. It occurs more frequently in areas with low or deficient selenium concentration

24. **Congenital porphyria in cattle is an example of:**

a. Primary photosensitization

b. Hepatogenous photosensitization

c. Photosensitivity of unknown aetiology

d. Photosensitivity due to aberrant pigment synthesis

25. **Which of the following is not a secondary morphologic skin lesion?**

    a. Ulcer

    b. Lichenification

    c. Purpura

    d. Fissure

26. **Concerning photosensitization, which of the following statements is correct?**

    a. It is a normal cutaneous reaction to UV

    b. In hepatic photosensitization, phylloerythrin accumulates in skin tissue

    c. In primary photosensitization, the liver produces photodynamic agents

    d. Photosensitization is a problem during the winter

27. **Which of the following is not a topical antifungal?**

    a. Chlorhexidine

    b. Povidone iodine

    c. Miconazole

    d. Silver-sulphadiazine

28. **Which of the following corresponds to 'sheep itch mites'?**

    a. Psorergatic mange

    b. Sarcoptic mange

    c. Psoroptic mange

    d. Chorioptic mange

29. **Serum elevation of which enzyme is a good indication of active muscle damage?**

    a. CPK

    b. AST

    c. ALT

    d. AP

30. **In meningoencephalitis, the following changes are seen in CSF, except:**

    a. Increased protein content

    b. Increased number of neutrophils

    c. Increased number of lymphocytes

    d. Reticulocytosis

31. **A factor commonly leading to exertional myopathy in horses is:**

    a. Protein deficient diet

    b. Hyperkalemic periodic paralysis

    c. Chronic laminitis

    d. Change in exercise pattern

32. **Which of the following antimicrobials is effective against betalactamase-producing anaerobic bacteria?**

    a. Penicillin

    b. Cephalexin

    c. Ceftiofur

    d. Metronidazole

33. **Deficiency of which of the following is associated with the feeding of a large quantity of uncooked fish?**

    a. Pantothenic acid

    b. Thiamine

    c. Vitamin C

    d. Riboflavin

34. **Which of the following is commonly associated with the granulomatous type of meningitis?**

    a. *Cryptococcus neoformis*

    b. *Aspergillus flavus*

    c. *Histoplasma farciminosum*

    d. *Histoplasma capsulatum*

35. **Leukoencephalomalacia in horses is characterized by:**

    a. Aimless wandering and head pressing

    b. Paralysis, dysuriaparesis and hyperexcitability

    c. Blindness and pupillary dilatation

    d. Depression, facial paralysis and circling

36. **Fever with enlarged superficial lymph nodes in cross-bred calves is usually seen in:**

    a. Coccidiomycosis

    b. Piroplasmosis

    c. Theileriosis

    d. Toxoplasmosis

37. **Which of the following is not a sequalae of FMD?**

    a. Infertility

    b. Panting

    c. Deformities of hooves

    d. Myocarditis

38. **Which of the following is not a differential of hypomagnesemic tetany in cattle?**

    a. Acute lead poisoning

    b. Rabies

    c. BSE

    d. Stagger syndrome

39. **Deg-Nala disease is associated with:**

    a. Deprivation

    b. Mouldy rice straw

    c. Vitamin E/selenium toxicity

    d. Cu poisoning

40. **Which clinicopathologic finding is not compatible with ketosis in ruminants?**

    a. Hypoglycaemia

    b. Ketonemia

    c. Ketonuria

    d. Hypocalcaemia

41. **Determination of the concentration of blood urea nitrogen provides a crude index of:**

    a. Renal tubular secretory capacity

    b. Renal tubular reabsorptive capacity

    c. Glomerular filtration rate

    d. Renal plasma flow

42. **Impetigo is a superficial pustular dermatitis that usually begins on the:**

    a. Lips

    b. Ears

    c. Udder

    d. Back

43. **A surf field mastitis test (a screening test) to access the leukocyte count in milk, and treatment to remove the organism from the infected udder before the signs of mastitis develop are examples of:**

    a. Primary prevention

    b. Secondary prevention

    c. Eradication

    d. Vector control

44. **The capacity of an agent to cause disease in a susceptible host is defined as:**

    a. Virulence

    b. Pathogenicity

c. Infectivity

d. Aggressiveness

45. **An infection that results in no noticeable clinical signs is called a:**

a. Clinical infection

b. Convalescent infection

c. Dead-end infection

d. Inapparent infection

46. **The species in which an organism is maintained is called a:**

a. Carrier

b. Vector

c. Source

d. Reservoir

47. **The place from which an infectious agent passes directly to a susceptible host is known as the:**

a. Source

b. Reservoir

c. Portal of entry

d. Vehicle

48. **The proportion of diseased animals in a population at a given time is known as the:**

a. Incidence

b. Attack rate

c. Prevalence

d. Point prevalence

49. **Which of the following is not an example of direct transmission of an infectious agent?**

a. Aerosol transmission

b. Venereal transmission

    c. Foodborne transmission

    d. Horizontal transmission

50. **Which of the following is the least likely to aid in management and prevention of haemorrhagic septicemia?**

    a. Increasing ventilation rate

    b. Maintaining shed temperature between 32–35°C

    c. Reducing animal density

    d. Decreasing shed humidity to 50%

51. ***Mycobacterium tuberculosis*, the usual cause of human tuberculosis:**

    a. Can infect bovines

    b. Infects only people

    c. Has limited host range

    d. Is typically destroyed by human saliva

52. **What is the most appropriate action for a case of anthrax in a cow?**

    a. Don't report the disease to the animal disease authorities

    b. Vaccinate all food animals against anthrax

    c. Always perform a complete necropsy

    d. Bury/or burn the carcass as soon as possible after diagnosis

53. **The most common source of listeriosis in sheep is:**

    a. Environmental contamination

    b. Contaminated water

    c. Contaminated hay

    d. Spoiled silage

54. **Enterotoxaemia is a deadly ovine disease best controlled by vaccination and:**

    a. Addition of antibiotics to feed

    b. Proper nutritional management

    c. Feeding a high grain diet

    d. Periodic injection of selenium

55. **Differential diagnosis of weight loss in small ruminants includes all of the following except:**

    a. Caseous lymphadenitis

    b. Chronic hemoncosis

    c. Johne's disease

    d. Toxoplasmosis

56. **Antibacterial therapy of sheep with enterotoxaemia:**

    a. Should be given before initiation of fluid therapy

    b. Should be in the form of an oral solution rather than a tablet

    c. Should be administered parenterally

    d. Should be followed by oral administration of yoghurt to re-establish the intestinal flora

57. **'Sulphur granules' can be seen in the following conditions, except:**

    a. Actinobacillosis

    b. Actinomycosis

    c. Staphylococcal infection

    d. Sporotrichosis

58. **The treatment of black leg involves the following, except:**

    a. Administration of penicillin

    b. Surgical debulking and fenestration of lesion

    c. Administration of specific antitoxins

    d. Intralesional injection of BCG

59. **Differential diagnosis of anthrax includes the following, except:**

    a. Peracute black leg

    b. Malignant oedema

c. Lightning stroke

d. BSE

60. **Which condition is most likely to be confused with equine tetanus?**

a. White muscle disease

b. Polioencephalomalacia

c. Hyperkalemic periodic paralysis

d. Myotonia congenita

61. **In anthrax control, the following measures must be implemented, except:**

a. Correct disposal of the carcass

b. Correct disinfection, decontamination and disposal of contaminated materials

c. Vaccination of exposed susceptible animals and humans in at-risk occupations

d. Bathing of healthy animals with a mixture of 1% formaldehyde and 3% glutaraldehyde

62. **Which of the following is not a differential diagnosis of black disease?**

a. Acute leptospirosis

b. Post parturient hemoglobinuria

c. Chronic Cu poisoning

d. Anaplasmosis

63. **Chronic molybdenum poisoning in cattle is likely to be confused with:**

a. Johne's disease

b. Polyarthritis

c. Actinomycosis

d. Bacillary hemoglobinuria

64. **Which of the following drugs is not suitable for the treatment of actinobacillosis in buffalo?**

    a. Sodium iodide

    b. Isoniazid

    c. Lincomycin

    d. Ulphadiazine + trimethoprim

65. **Which of the following is an infectious but not a contagious disease?**

    a. Leptospirosis

    b. Tetanus

    c. Brucellosis

    d. Mucosal disease complex

66. **Equine glanders is caused by:**

    a. *Burkholderia mallei*

    b. *Burkholderia pseudomallei*

    c. *Burkholderia capaciae*

    d. *Burkholderia tialendesis*

67. **Which of the following antibiotics is not effective against *Mycoplasma*?**

    a. Penicillin

    b. Tylosin

    c. Gentamycin

    d. Oxytetracycline

68. **Nosocomial infections are:**

    a. Fatal infections

    b. Moderate infections

    c. Hospital acquired infections

    d. Infections acquired through the nostrils

69. **Superinfection refers to:**

    a. Fatal infections

    b. Moderate infections

    c. Secondary infections superimposing a less severe infection

    d. Secondary infections caused by yeast

70. **'Blitz therapy' in the context of treatment of *Streptococcus agalactiae* mastitis refers to:**

    a. Use of drugs which produce blisters on the udder

    b. Treatment of all lactating animals with penicillin

    c. Intramammary + intravenous treatment

    d. Use of antibiotics with corticosteroids

71. **In ruminal lactic acidosis, the following changes are seen in the rumen except:**

    a. *Streptococcus bovis* increases markedly

    b. The rumen pH falls below 5

    c. Depletion of lactate utilizing organism

    d. Destruction of *Lactobacilli*

72. **All but one of these is not a pathophysiological consequence of ruminal lactic acidosis. Which one?**

    a. Haemoconcentration

    b. Renal failure

    c. Muscular weakness

    d. Increased urine pH

73. **A synonym of traumatic reticuloperitonitis is:**

    a. Rumen impaction

    b. Grain overload

    c. Hardware disease

    d. Ruminal tympany

74. **Concerning ruminal tympany, which of the following is incorrect?**

    a. Bloat is a common cause of sudden death

    b. Susceptibility of cattle to bloat is genetically determined

    c. Disease is associated with drought

    d. Cessation of respiration is the cause of death

75. **Which of the following is a reportable disease?**

    a. Glanders

    b. Degnala

    c. Tetanus

    d. Strangles

76. **Indirect bilirubin in the serum is the indication of what?**

    a. Haemolytic jaundice

    b. Hepatic jaundice

    c. Obstructive jaundice

    d. Toxic jaundice

77. **What is the most common skin tumour affecting horses?**

    a. Squamous cell carcinoma

    b. Viral papitomatosis

    c. Basal cell carcinoma

    d. Melanoma

78. **Horse sickness fever is mostly observed in:**

    a. Donkeys

    b. Zebras

    c. Immunized horses

    d. All of above

79. **Equine infectious anaemia has:**

    a. 1 form

    b. 2 forms

c. 3 forms

d. 4 forms

80. **The natural vector of equine infectious anaemia is:**

a. Stable fly

b. Deer fly

c. Horse fly

d. Mosquito

81. **In rabies in horses, ascending paralysis develops:**

a. In furious form

b. In dumb form

c. a and b

d. None of these

82. **Countries free of rabies maintain this status by:**

a. Vaccination

b. Quarantine

c. a and b

d. None of these

83. **Vascular stomatitis is characterized by:**

a. Vesicles on the feet

b. Vesicles in the mouth

c. Vesicles on the feet and in the mouth

d. Vesicles on the abdomen

84. **Arboviruses are transmitted by:**

a. Arthropods

b. Inhalation

c. Ingestion

d. Congenital transmission

85. **Diarrhoeal illness in foals is caused by:**

    a. Herpes virus

    b. Rota virus

    c. Equine influenza virus

    d. Alpha virus

86. **Foals acquire the *Actinobacillus equuli* organism:**

    a. From their surroundings

    b. In utero

    c. Soon after birth

    d. All of above

87. **In salmonellosis, young foals die due to:**

    a. Hypovolemic shock

    b. Septic shock

    c. Diarrhoea

    d. Respiratory collapse

88. **Enterotoxaemia in new-born foals is associated with *Clostridium perfringens* type:**

    a. A

    b. B

    c. C

    d. B and C

89. **The causative agent of *Rhodococcus equi* is localized in:**

    a. Joints

    b. Respiratory tract

    c. Gastrointestinal tract

    d. a and c

90. **Dermatophilosis is also referred to as:**

    a. Subcutaneous streptothricosis

    b. Rain scald

c. Mud fever

d. All of above

91. Clostridial necrotizing cellulitis is also called:

a. Wound gas gangrene

b. Malignant oedema

c. Myositis

d. All of these

92. Toxicoinfectious botulism is known to occur in:

a. Horses

b. Humans

c. Horses and humans

d. None of these

93. Shaker foal syndrome is a form of:

a. Spontaneous toxicoinfectious botulism

b. Toxicoinfectious botulism

c. a and b

d. None of these

94. Clinical signs of tetanus are indicated by:

a. Tetanospasmin

b. Interaction between tetanospasmin and nervous tissue

c. Damage to nervous tissue

d. Tetanolysin

95. Haemorrhagic necrosis and gross swelling of all lymphoid organs in horses is seen in:

a. Glanders

b. Anthrax

c. Tetanus

d. Strangles

96. **Streptococcal infection is most common in:**

   a. Older horses

   b. Young horses

   c. Neonates

   d. a and b

97. **In foals, pigeon fever is the name given to abscesses in the form of:**

   a. *Corynebacterium pseudotuberculosis*

   b. *Histoplasma farciminosum*

   c. Melioidosis

   d. None of these

98. **Which are the major pinworms in horses?**

   a. *Parascaris equorum*

   b. *Oxyuris equi*

   c. *Gastrophilus*

   d. *Anoplocephala*

99. **Which are the major tapeworms in horses?**

   a. *Gastrophilus*

   b. *Parascaris equorum*

   c. *Anoplocephala*

   d. *Strongyloides westeri*

100. **'Horse bots' are:**

   a. *Gastrophilus*

   b. *Oxyuris equi*

   c. *Parascaris equorum*

   d. *Dictyocaulus arnfieldi*

101. **Which are the major roundworms in horses?**

a. *Parascaris equorum*

b. *Strongylus vulgaris*

c. *Triodontophorus*

d. *Cyathostomum*

102. **Which are the major lungworms in horses?**

a. *Anoplocephala species*

b. *Gastrophilus species*

c. *Parascaris equorum*

d. *Dictyocaulus arnfieldi*

103. **Which are the major threadworms in horses?**

a. *Strongylus vulgaris*

b. *Strongylus westeri*

c. *Oxyuris equi*

d. *Dictyocaulus arnfieldi*

104. **Which *Trypanosome* species is not involved in nagana in horses?**

a. *T. Congolense*

b. *T. brucei*

c. *T. vivax*

d. *T. evansi*

105. **Which *Trypanosome* is not involved in surra in horses?**

a. *T. equinum*

b. *T. evansi*

c. *T. vivax*

d. None of these are involved

106. **Which *Trypanosome* is involved in dourine in horses?**

a. *T. equiperdum*

b. *T. evansi*

c. *T. equinum*

d. *T. brucei*

107. **Dourine *Trypanosome* in horses is transmitted by:**

a. Biting flies

b. Tsetse flies

c. Vampire bats

d. Coitus

108. **Which of the following are trypanocidal drugs in horses?**

a. Febantal

b. Quinapyramine

c. Suramin

d. b and c

109. **Imidocarb is used in horses for:**

a. Babesiosis

b. Trypanosomiasis

c. Fascioliasis

d. Hydatidosis

110. **The drug of choice in habronemiasis in horses is:**

a. Diminazine

b. Ivermectin

c. Suramin

d. Imidocarb

111. **Which of the following is a flukicidal drug in horses?**

a. Buparvaquone

b. Imidocarb

c. Rafoxanide

d. Diminazine

112. **Periodic ophthalmia is seen in horses with:**
    a. Leptospirosis
    b. Ehrlichiosis
    c. Melioidosis
    d. b and c

113. **In horses, leptospirosis is mostly transmitted by:**
    a. Faeces
    b. Water
    c. Urine
    d. a and c

114. **Meliodosis in horses is caused by:**
    a. *Pseudomonas pseudomallei*
    b. *Ehrlichia risticii*
    c. *Ehrlichia equi*
    d. None of these

115. **One of the most ancient diseases recognized in horses is:**
    a. Strangles
    b. Glanders
    c. Meliodosis
    d. Ehrlichiosis

116. **Glanders in horses is caused by:**
    a. *Pseudomonas pseudomallei*
    b. *Pseudomonas aeruginosa*
    c. *Pseudomonas mallei*
    d. a and c

117. **Mallein is a protein produced by:**
    a. *Pseudomonas mallei*
    b. *Pseudomonas pseudomallei*

    c. *Pseudomonas aeruginosa*

    d. a and b

118. **In horses, folliculitis is also called:**

    a. Canadian horse pox

    b. Dry land distemper

    c. Colorado distemper

    d. b and c

119. **In horses, the inability to retract the nictitating membrane is seen in:**

    a. Tetanus

    b. Anthrax

    c. Glanders

    d. Strangles

120. **Forage poisoning in horses is caused by *Clostridium* type:**

    a. A

    b. B

    c. A and B

    d. C

121. **In equines, the *Clostridium* not involved in necrotizing cellulites is:**

    a. *Cl. perfringens*

    b. *Cl. novyi*

    c. *Cl. septicum*

    d. *Cl. botulinum*

122. **Equine distemper is also referred to as:**

    a. Equine viral arteritis

    b. Glanders

    c. Strangles

    d. Equine influenza

123. **In horses, ringworm infection is also called:**

    a. Cryptococcosis

    b. Histoplasmosis

    c. Dermatomycosis

    d. Rhinosporidiosis

124. **Thrombocytopenia is common in horses with:**

    a. Ehrlichiosis

    b. Histoplasmosis

    c. Sporotrichosis

    d. Blastomycosis

125. **Equine infectious anaemia is also called:**

    a. Wanderer's

    b. Swamp fever

    c. Barker's

    d. None of these

126. **African horse sickness is:**

    a. Infectious

    b. Contagious

    c. Infectious and contagious

    d. None of these

127. **Equine influenza virus is transmitted by which route?**

    a. Inhalation

    b. Ingestion

    c. Congenital

    d. a and b

128. **The cause of flatulent colic in horses is:**

    a. Simple obstruction of the intestinal lumen

    b. Excessive gas in the intestinal lumen

    c. A strangulating obstruction

    d. Enteritis

129. The anthelmintic not associated with ascarid impaction in horses is:

    a. Ivermectin

    b. Benzimidazole

    c. Piperazine

    d. Organophosphate

130. Equine herpesvirus infection is also called:

    a. Equine abortion virus

    b. Equine arteritis

    c. Equine rhinopneumonitis

    d. None of these

131. Equine abortion virus infection is also called:

    a. Equine herpesvirus

    b. Equine arteritis

    c. Equine rhinopneumonitis

    d. None of these

132. The most serious cause of pneumonia in foals is:

    a. *Streptococcus equi*

    b. *Rhodococcus equi*

    c. *Streptococcus equi equi*

    d. a and c

133. In horses, guttural pouch empyema is caused by:

    a. *Staphylococcus*

    b. *Streptococcus*

    c. *Pseudomonas*

    d. *Clostridium*

134. **The primary cause of ringworm in horses is:**

    a. *Microsporum gypseum*

    b. *Microsporum canis*

    c. *Trichophyton equinum*

    d. *Trichophyton verrucosum*

135. **In horses, arboviruses are transmitted by:**

    a. Mosquitoes

    b. Flies

    c. Vampire bats

    d. Ticks

136. **In horses, the cause of heave line is:**

    a. Heaves

    b. Chronic obstructive pulmonary disease

    c. Equine influenza

    d. a and b

137. **Potomac horse fever is caused by:**

    a. *Neorickettsia risticii*

    b. *Ehrlichia equi*

    c. *Pseudomonas aeruginosa*

    d. None of these

138. **Colibacillosis in horses is caused by:**

    a. *Klebsiella*

    b. *Escherichia coli*

    c. *Pseudomonas aeruginosa*

    d. *Salmonella typhimurium*

139. ***Salmonella* in horses is transmitted by:**

    a. Flies

    b. Contaminated feed and water

    c. Carrier horses

    d. All of these

140. Which stain is used for confirmation of Tyzzer's disease in horses?

    a. Giemsa

    b. Warthin-Starry

    c. Gram

    d. a and b

141. In horses, tetanus toxin is distributed by:

    a. 3 routes

    b. 2 routes

    c. 4 routes

    d. Multiple routes

142. In equine tetanus, antitoxin is injected by:

    a. Muscular route

    b. Intravenous route

    c. Intradermal route

    d. Subarachnoid space

143. The anthrax organism is very sensitive to:

    a. Penicillin

    b. Tetracyclines

    c. Aminoglycosides

    d. a and b

144. Pyogenic dermatitis in horses is caused by:

    a. *Streptococcus*

    b. *Staphylococcus*

    c. *Pseudomonas*

    d. *Salmonella*

145. **Diagnosis of 'poll evil' is confirmed by isolating *B. abortus* from:**

   a. Blood

   b. Bursa

   c. Nasal discharge

   d. None of these

146. **In horse listeriosis, the drug of choice is:**

   a. Oxytetracycline

   b. Penicillin

   c. Aminoglycoside

   d. All of these

147. **The most frequently encountered pyogen in horses is:**

   a. *Staphylococcus aureus*

   b. *Pseudomonas aeruginosa*

   c. *Escherichia coli*

   d. *Streptococcus zooepidemicus*

148. **In horse bots, ivermectin is effective against:**

   a. Oral stages

   b. Gastric stages

   c. Pulmonary stages

   d. a and b

149. **Cyathomostomiasis is a condition in horses associated with:**

   a. Small strongyles

   b. Large strongyles

   c. Pinworms

   d. Stomach bots

150. **In horses, pyrantel is not effective against:**

   a. *Oxyuris equi*

   b. Large strongyles

c. *Parascaris equorum*

d. *Strongyloides westeri*

151. **Thiabendazole is not effective against:**

a. Stomach bots

b. *Oxyuris equi*

c. Large strongyles

d. Small strongyles

152. **The drug recommended for lungworm infection in horses is:**

a. Mebendazole

b. Ivermectin

c. Pyrantel

d. Febantel

153. **The drug recommended for tapeworm infection in horses is:**

a. Pyrantel

b. Ivermectin

c. Oxyclozanide

d. Febantal

154. **A common cause of unthriftiness in foals is:**

a. Strongyloidosis

b. Parascariasis

c. Lungworm infection

d. All of these

155. **Reproductive tract disease in mares is caused by:**

a. *Klebsiella pneumoniae*

b. *Pseudomonas aeruginosa*

c. *Streptococcus equi*

d. *Escherichia coli*

156. In horses, oxfendazole is not effective against:

a. *Parascaris equorum*

b. *Oxyuris equi*

c. Stomach bots

d. Large strongyles

157. A broad spectrum anthelmintic used in horses is:

a. Thiabendazole

b. Febantel

c. Pyrantel

d. Ivermectin

158. Determination of the seat and nature of disease is known as:

a. Diagnosis

b. History

c. Clinical examination

d. Physical examination

159. The probable outcome of a disease is known as:

a. Recovery

b. Prognosis

c. Tentative diagnosis

d. Sequelae

160. The treatment directed towards the cause of a disease is known as:

a. Symptomatic treatment

b. Supportive treatment

c. Treatment complication

d. Specific treatment

161. **Measures to prevent the spread of a disease when it is likely to develop in animals is known as:**

    a. Empirical treatment

    b. Metaphylactic treatment

    c. Non-specific treatment

    d. Prophylactic treatment

162. **Pyrogenic stimulation of the thermoregulatory centre is known as:**

    a. Hypothermia

    b. Heatstroke

    c. Fever

    d. Heat prostration

163. **The most common exogenous toxin of G-ve bacteria is:**

    a. Lipid-A

    b. Lipid-B

    c. Lipid-D

    d. Lipid-E

164. **A drug frequently used to treat collapse or shock is:**

    a. Dipyron

    b. Salicylic acid

    c. Steroid

    d. Phenylbutazone

165. **Depression of nervous activity and respiratory centre occurs at which critical temperature (Fahrenheit):**

    a. 102

    b. 103

    c. 105

    d. Above 108

166. **Ruminants and pet mammals are more prone to hyperthermia due to:**

    a. Less sweat glands

    b. More sweat glands

    c. No sweat glands

    d. Thick coat

167. **The 'horseshoe crab' amoebocytes test is used for determination of:**

    a. Endotoxin toxin

    b. Bacteria

    c. Virus

    d. Uric acid

168. **Type-II hypersensitivity reaction is produced due to:**

    a. IgG

    b. IgM

    c. IgG and IgM

    d. IgD

169. **For treatment of anaphylactic shock, the first drug of choice is:**

    a. Dexamethasone

    b. Adrenaline

    c. Prednisolone

    d. Cortisone

170. **Stomatitis is a common condition in diseases such as:**

    a. Actinobacillosis

    b. HS

    c. Black quarter

    d. Flu

171. **Hypersalivation can be controlled by:**

    a. Boric acid

    b. Glycerine

    c. Atropine sulphate

    d. Lignocain

172. **A common complication of pharyngitis is:**

    a. Bronchitis

    b. Laryngitis

    c. Aspiratory pneumonia

    d. Tracheitis

173. **The number-one cause of death in horses is:**

    a. Strangles

    b. Colic

    c. Gastritis

    d. Glanders

174. **Bacterial toxin induces vomiting by stimulating:**

    a. CRTZ

    b. Higher brain

    c. VA

    d. PSR

175. **During vomiting, the most frequent electrolyte abnormality is deficiency of what?**

    a. Na

    b. K

    c. HCO_3

    d. Cl

176. **Which of the following is an example of a centrally acting antiemetic?**

   a. Phenothiazine

   b. Diphenhydramine

   c. Meclizine

   d. Avil

177. **Which is an example of broad-spectrum antiemetic?**

   a. Metacloperamide

   b. Dimenhydrinate

   c. Phenothiazine

   d. Trimethobenzamide

178. **Colic due to torsion and strangulation of the intestine is known as:**

   a. Spasmodic

   b. Impactive

   c. Obstructive

   d. Idiopathic

179. **The cause of death in colic may be rupture of the:**

   a. Stomach

   b. Abdomen cavity

   c. Oesophagus

   d. Pharynx

180. **Antispasmodic drugs used to treat spasmodic colic include:**

   a. Atropine sulphate

   b. Metoclopramide

   c. Neostigmine

   d. All of these

181.   In acute flatulent colic, an emergency measure is to use:

a. Stomach powder

b. Vegetables

c. Trocar and canula

d. Purgatives

182.   In diarrhoea and dehydration, loss of H+ can lead to:

a. Hypoglycemia

b. Acidosis

c. Alkalosis

d. None of these

183.   A fishy smell of faeces indicates decomposition of:

a. Fat

b. Cellulose

c. Protein

d. None of these

184.   A pungent smell of faeces is diagnostic of:

a. TB

b. FMD

c. PPR

d. Salmonellosis

185.   An offensive odour of faeces is diagnostic of:

a. Abnormal fermentation

b. Protein decomposition

c. Pancreatic insufficiency

d. All of these

186.   Which critical loss of body fluid causes death?

a. 4%

b. 5%

c. 6%

d. 10%

187. **In severe acidosis, what percentage of bicarbonate solution should be used?**

a. 1.3%

b. 5%

c. 7.5%

d. 9%

188. **A sedimentation activity test is used for diagnosing:**

a. Diarrhoea

b. Simple indigestion

c. Tympany

d. All of these

189. **Rumenitoric drugs such as 'Nux Vomica' are recommended for:**

a. GIT disturbance

b. Colic

c. Pyrexia

d. All of these

190. **Antizymotic drugs are indicated in:**

a. Gastritis

b. Tympany

c. Enteritis

d. Diarrhoea

191. **If ingested by animals, plants containing pectin and saponin can lead to:**

a. Gastritis

b. Tympany

c. Bloat

d. None of these

192. **A case of 'foreign body' in ruminants can be diagnosed by:**

a. Ultrasound

b. X-rays

c. Metal detector

d. All of the above

193. **Excessive ingestion of grains by animals can lead to:**

a. Rumen impaction

b. Acidosis

c. Diarrhoea

d. All of these

194. **Which of the following is a site for measurement of pulse rate in cattle?**

a. Facial artery

b. Middle coccygeal artery

c. Facial and middle coccygeal arteries

d. None of these

195. **In foals, joint illness develops due to:**

a. Umbilicus infection

b. Localization of organism in joints

c. Inflammation of tendons

d. Delayed intake of colostrum

196. **In horses, neonatal maladjustment syndrome is also known as:**

a. Wanderers

b. Barkers

c. Heaves

d. a and b

197. **Combined immunodeficiency disease is also known as:**

a. Neonatal isoerythrolysis

b. Dummies

   c. Convulsive foals

   d. None of these

198. A disease of Arabian or part-Arabian foals is:

   a. Dummies

   b. 'Convulsive foals'

   c. Combined immunodeficiency disease

   d. Neonatal isoerythrolysis

199. How many types of equine herpesvirus are there?

   a. 5

   b. 4

   c. 3

   d. 2

200. Adenovirus infection is the most prevalent cause of death in Arabian foals with:

   a. Combined immuno-deficiency

   b. Dummies

   c. Barkers

   d. Heaves

201. African horse sickness has how many forms?

   a. 5

   b. 3

   c. 4

   d. 1

202. The mildest form of African horse sickness is:

   a. Sub-acute or cardiac

   b. Mixed

   c. Acute or pulmonary

   d. Horse sickness fever

203. **The most common type of urinary calculi found in bovines is:**

    a. Phosphate

    b. Silicate

    c. Sulfate

    d. Carbonate

204. **Pylonephritis in cattle is commonly caused by:**

    a. *E. coli*

    b. *Corynebacterium pyogenes*

    c. *Pseudomonas aeruginosa*

    d. *Corynebacterium renale*

205. **One of the non-benzimidazole derivative anthelmintics is:**

    a. Febantel

    b. Fenbendazole

    c. Miconazole

    d. Natamycin

206. **Tyzzer's disease is caused by:**

    a. *Bacillus piliformis*

    b. *Rhodococcus equi*

    c. *Salmonella typhimurium*

    d. *Actinobacillus equuli*

207. **Obstructive pulmonary disease is also referred to as:**

    a. Cryptococcal respiratory infection

    b. Aspiration pneumonia

    c. Smoke inhalation injury

    d. Chronic alveolar emphysema

208. **Gastric squamous cell carcinoma is diagnosed by:**

    a. Contrast radiography

    b. Exploratory laparotomy

c. Fibreoptoscopic examination

d. Neoplastic squamous cells in pleural fluid

209. **Cystitis is usually accompanied by:**

a. Urethritis

b. Nephritis

c. Nephrosis

d. Urolithiasis

210. **Haemoglobinuria is associated with:**

a. Tubular nephrosis

b. Glomerular nephrosis

c. Hydronephrosis

d. b and c

211. **Normal urine in horses is:**

a. Opaque

b. Turbid

c. Clear

d. a and b

212. **In horses, tachycardia is common in:**

a. Pneumonia

b. Metabolic acidosis

c. Haemolytic disease

d. Atelectasis

213. **A causal organism in younger foal infections is:**

a. *Streptococci*

b. *Klebsiella*

c. *Salmonella*

d. *Corynebacterium*

214. **Actinobacillus equuli is found in the:**

a. Respiratory tract

b. Gastrointestinal tract

c. Reproductive tract

d. None of these

215. **In foals, joint illness develops due to:**

a. Umbilicus infection

b. Localization of causative organism in joints

c. Inflammation of tendons

d. Delayed intake of colostrum

216. **In horses, neonatal maladjustment syndrome is also known as:**

a. Wanderers

b. Barkers

c. Heaves

d. a and b

217. **Combined immunodeficiency disease is also known as:**

a. Neonatal isoerythrolysis

b. Dummies

c. Convulsive foals

d. None of these

218. **Accumulation of air in the chest is known as:**

a. Pneumonia

b. Pneumonitis

c. Chylothorax

d. Pneumothorax

219. **Neoplasia of the spleen is best treated by:**

a. Splenectomy

b. Chemotherapy

c. Irradiation

d. No treatment

220. **Which one of the following conditions is not an indication for spaying?**

a. Pseudocyesis

b. Nymphomania

c. Mammary tumours

d. Gynecomastia

221. **The best age for a mature female dog to have an ovario-hysterectomy is:**

a. First day of oestrus

b. Last day of oestrus

c. 2 to 3 days after parturition

d. 6 to 8 weeks after parturition

222. **The cause of pseudoestrus in ovariohysterectomized female dogs is:**

a. Chronic vaginitis

b. Metritis

c. Salpingitis

d. Oophritis

223. **Intra-arterial injection for splenic contraction during splenectomy is contraindicated in cases of:**

a. Splenic torsion

b. Hypersplenism

c. Splenomegaly

d. Splenic neoplasms

224. **Where do alimentary foreign bodies most commonly lodge?**

a. Pharyngeal oesophagus

b. Oesophagus near the base of the heart

c. Oesophagus in the diaphragmatic vital region

d. Duodenum

225. **What type of system is most effective for draining an effusion associated with generalized peritonitis?**

a. Closed suction drain

b. Continuous suction drain

c. Open peritoneal drainage

d. Penrose drain

226. **What is the primary treatment for acute elbow hygroma?**

a. Providing a well-padded area

b. Aseptically draining of hygroma

c. Excision of affected area

d. Oral corticosteroid and antibiotics

227. **Castration can be used in treatment or prevention of all the following disorders except:**

a. Perianal fistula

b. Perianal adenoma

c. Chronic prostalitis

d. Benign prostatic hyperplasia

228. **What is an isograft?**

a. A graft in which the donor tissue is not of the same organ type as the recipient

b. A graft in which tissue is transferred to a new position on the same individual

c. A graft in which the donor and recipient are different individuals but genetically identical

d. A graft in which the donor and recipient are genetically not identical

229. **The mucocoele developed in salivary glands are known as:**

a. Sailocoele

b. Hydrocoele

c. Angiocoele

d. Salivary nidus

230. **The term used to describe a salivary mucocoele located ventral to the tongue is:**

a. Ranula

b. Lingnoma

c. Cyst

d. Cavity

231. **Which wound is most prone to anaerobic infection?**

a. Contusion

b. Laceration

c. Incision

d. Puncture

232. **The most common cryogenic agent used in veterinary medicine is:**

a. Liquid nitrogen

b. Dry ice

c. Freon

d. Nitrous oxide

233. **Lithotripsy is used to treat what?**

a. Faecolith

b. Urolith

c. Sailolith

d. Gallstones

Answers

1.	a	31.	d	61.	c	91.	a
2.	b	32.	a	62.	d	92.	a
3.	b	33.	b	63.	d	93.	c
4.	b	34.	a	64.	d	94.	a
5.	b	35.	a	65.	b	95.	b
6.	d	36.	c	66.	a	96.	d
7.	a	37.	a	67.	b	97.	a
8.	c	38.	c	68.	c	98.	b
9.	a	39.	b	69.	c	99.	c
10.	b	40.	d	70.	c	100.	a
11.	a	41.	c	71.	a	101.	a
12.	a	42.	c	72.	a	102.	d
13.	c	43.	a	73.	c	103.	c
14.	b	44.	b	74.	c	104.	d
15.	c	45.	b	75.	a	105.	a
16.	b	46.	d	76.	c	106.	a
17.	c	47.	c	77.	c	107.	d
18.	a	48.	a	78.	d	108.	d
19.	b	49.	b	79.	c	109.	a
20.	a	50.	a	80.	a	110.	b
21.	c	51.	a	81.	b	111.	c
22.	d	52.	d	82.	c	112.	d
23.	c	53.	c	83.	b	113.	d
24.	a	54.	b	84.	a	114.	a
25.	c	55.	a	85.	b	115.	b
26.	b	56.	c	86.	a	116.	c
27.	b	57.	b	87.	a	117.	a
28.	a	58.	b	88.	c	118.	a
29.	a	59.	b	89.	b	119.	a
30.	d	60.	b	90.	b	120.	d

(Continued)

121.	a	150.	d	179.	a	208.	d
122.	c	151.	a	180.	c	209.	c
123.	c	152.	b	181.	c	210.	b
124.	a	153.	a	182.	c	211.	b
125.	b	154.	d	183.	c	212.	c
126.	c	155.	a	184.	d	213.	c
127.	d	156.	c	185.	d	214.	b
128.	b	157.	d	186.	d	215.	a
129.	d	158.	a	187.	c	216.	a
130.	a	159.	d	188.	c	217.	a
131.	a	160.	d	189.	a	218.	d
132.	d	161.	d	190.	b	219.	a
133.	a	162.	c	191.	c	220.	c
134.	c	163.	a	192.	d	221.	d
135.	b	164.	c	193.	d	222.	d
136.	d	165.	d	194.	b	223.	a
137.	a	166.	c	195.	a	224.	b
138.	b	167.	a	196.	d	225.	a
139.	d	168.	c	197.	d	226.	b
140.	b	169.	a	198.	c	227.	a
141.	d	170.	a	199.	c	228.	d
142.	a	171.	c	200.	a	229.	a
143.	d	172.	b	201.	c	230.	a
144.	b	173.	b	202.	d	231.	d
145.	d	174.	a	203.	a	232.	a
146.	b	175.	b	204.	d	233.	d
147.	a	176.	a	205.	c		
148.	d	177.	a	206.	a		
149.	b	178.	c	207.	d		

2 Clinical Examination

Neha Rao

Introduction

Clinical examination of animals is a crucial aspect of veterinary practice that helps in the diagnosis of various diseases and conditions. The diagnosis, treatment and control of diseases of farm animals is heavily dependent on the clinical examination of animals, and astute assessment of the environment and management practices. Veterinarians must be highly skilled in obtaining an accurate and useful clinical history and in conducting an adequate clinical examination to make an accurate diagnosis. The veterinarian uses the physical diagnostic skills of visual observation, auscultation, palpation, percussion, succession, ballottement and so on. Recent clinical disease history and clinical findings are much more powerful diagnostically than relying on laboratory data. It is important that the clinical examination should be carefully and thoughtfully carried out so that all clinically significant abnormalities can be detected. Systemic clinical examination provides valuable information about the animal's overall health status and helps the veterinarian to identify any illnesses or abnormalities.

Examination and Assessment

The first step in conducting a physical examination of an animal is taking a **history**. This involves gathering information about the animal's symptoms, the duration of the illness, and any previous treatments that have been carried out. History-taking is an important aspect of the examination as it helps the veterinarian to locate the disease and determine its potential causes.

Identification of the animal is the first step in conducting a physical examination. It is important to identify the species, sex, age, colour, colour markings, polledness and other identifying marks.

© CAB International 2024. *Key Questions in Clinical Farm Animal Medicine Volume 1: Principles of Disease Examination, Diagnosis and Management* (ed. T. Rana)
DOI: 10.1079/9781800624788.0002

Good **communication skills** are an essential component of successful history-taking. The use of non-technical terms is usually essential, because livestock owners can be confused by technical expressions or reluctant to express themselves when confronted with terms they do not understand. The veterinarian must be aware of the vernacular associated with particular breeds or uses of animals and should be able to communicate in these terms.

History-taking will vary considerably depending on whether one animal or a group of animals in a herd are being examined. Attempts should be made to elicit the details of the clinical abnormalities of present illness in a sequential manner. If more than one animal is affected, a typical case should be chosen and the variations in history in other cases should then be noted. Variations from the norm in the physiologic functions, such as intake of food or water, milk production, growth, respiration, defecation, urination, sweating, activity, gait, posture, voice and odour should be noted in all cases. Morbidity, case fatality and population mortality rates must be recorded. Any prior treatment and prophylactic and control measures should be recorded.

Information elicited by questioning about previous history of illness can be helpful. If there is a history of previous illness, enquiries should be made along the usual lines, including clinical observations, necropsy findings, morbidity, case fatality rates, the treatments and control measures used, and the results obtained.

The **management history** includes nutrition, breeding policy and practice, housing, transport and so on. Breeding and parturition history may suggest or eliminate some diagnostic possibilities. Many diseases are influenced by climate (e.g. vector-borne diseases, a hot, humid climate). A general management history in relation to housing, feeding, watering, breeding and other practices should be taken. Any deviation from routine practices may provide clues for illness.

Examination of the environment

An examination of the environment is a necessary part of any clinical investigation because of the possible relationship between environmental factors and the incidence of disease. Some animals are raised indoors, whereas others are at pasture. The effects of topography, plants, soil type, ground surface and protection from extremes of weather assume major importance in animals raised at pasture. Similarly, for animals housed indoors, hygiene, ventilation, overcrowding and floor type are major factors.

Examination of the animal

Clinical examination is the focal point in any diagnostic process. More is missed by *not looking* than by *not knowing*. Clinical examinations aid in the identification of abnormalities in form and function of the animal, provide invaluable information regarding the cause of the disease, help to define the severity of the disease, and aid in monitoring the progression of the disease. A complete clinical examination of an animal includes, in addition to history-taking and examination of the environment, physical and laboratory examinations. The examination of an animal consists of a general inspection done from a distance, followed by a close physical examination of all body regions and systems.

General inspection is the most important part of clinical examination without disturbing the animal. Many observations such as behaviour, body condition and appearance, posture and gait can be recorded. Abnormalities in voice, prehension, mastication and swallowing – and, in ruminants, of belching and regurgitation – should be recorded. Urination and defecation should be noted. General body coat condition and skin abnormalities should be noted. Inspection of all the body parts from head to tail should be carried out.

Direct palpation with the fingers or **indirect palpation** with a probe is aimed at determining the size, consistency, temperature and sensitivity of a lesion or organ. Palpation of different organs may reveal the following conditions.

- *Doughy*: when the structure pits on pressure, as in oedema.
- *Firm*: when the structure has the consistency of a normal liver.
- *Hard*: when the consistency is bonelike.
- *Fluctuating*: when the structure is soft, elastic, and undulates on pressure but does not retain the imprint of the fingers, as in a cyst.
- *Tense*: when the structure feels like a viscus, distended with gas or fluid under some considerable pressure.
- *Emphysematous*: when the structure is puffy and swollen and moves and crackles under pressure because of the presence of gas in the tissue.

Percussion is the process of striking body parts to set deep parts in vibration and cause them to emit audible sounds. Percussion can be performed with the fingers using one hand as a plexor and one as a pleximeter. In large animals a pleximeter hammer on a pleximeter disc is recommended for consistency.

The sounds vary with the density of the parts set in vibration and may be classified as follows.

- *Resonant*: the sound emitted by organs containing air, as in a normal lung.
- *Tympanitic*: a drum-like note emitted by an organ containing gas under pressure, such as a tympanitic rumen or cecum.
- *Dull*: the sound emitted by solid organs such as the heart and liver.

Percussion is an important method in the diagnosis of diseases of the lungs and abdominal viscera of all large animals. Consolidation of the lung, pleural effusion or a space-occupying lesion, such as tumour or abscess, yields dull sound on percussion. Increased resonance over the thorax suggests emphysema or pneumothorax.

Ballottement is a modification of the palpation method to detect floating viscera or masses in the abdominal cavity. Using the extended fingers or the clenched fist, the abdominal wall is palpated with a firm push to displace the organ or mass, then allowing it to rebound on the fingertips.

Impaction of the abomasum, large tumours and abscesses of the abdominal cavity may also be detected by ballottement. Ballottement of a foetus is a typical example – the foetal prominences can be easily felt by pushing the gravid uterus through the abdominal wall over the right flank in pregnant cattle. Ballottement and auscultation of the left flank of cattle are also useful in detecting fluid-splashing sounds, as in ruminal acidosis. Over the right flank, fluid-splashing sounds may indicate intestinal obstruction, abomasal volvulus, caecal dilatation and torsion, and paralytic ileus.

A modification of the method is **tactile percussion,** when a cavity containing fluid is percussed sharply on one side and the fluid wave thus set up is palpated on the other. The sensation created by the fluid wave is called a 'fluid thrill', as in ascites and conditions causing fluid in the peritoneum.

Sounds produced by organs can be heard by **direct auscultation** – placing the ear to the body surface over the organ – or **indirect auscultation** – using a stethoscope is the preferred technique. Auscultation is used routinely to assess heart, lung and gastrointestinal sounds.

Percussion and simultaneous auscultation of the left and right sides of the abdomen is a useful technique for examination of the abdomen of large animals. This is a valuable diagnostic aid for the detection and localization of a gas-filled viscus in the abdomen of cattle with left-side displacement of the abomasum, right-side dilatation and volvulus of the abomasum, caecal dilatation and torsion, intestinal tympany associated with acute obstruction or paralytic ileus, or pneumoperitoneum.

To elicit the diagnostic 'ping', it is necessary to percuss and auscultate side by side and to percuss with a quick, sharp, light and localized force. A gas-filled viscus gives a characteristic clear, sharp, high-pitched ping, which is distinctly different from the full, low-pitched note of a solid or fluid-filled viscera.

Succussion involves moving the body from side to side to detect the presence of fluid. By performing careful auscultation while the body is moved, free fluid in the intestines or stomach will result in fluid splashing or tinkling sounds.

One of the most valuable adjuncts to a physical examination is a **radiographic examination** and **ultrasonography**. The size, location and shape of soft tissue organs are often demonstrable in animals of up to moderate size. Special physical techniques including **biopsy** and **paracentesis** are helpful in many conditions.

Sequence

Generally, an appropriate sequence for the close physical examination is as follows:

- *Vital signs*: temperature, heart and pulse rates, respirations and state of hydration.
- *Thorax*: heart sounds (rate, rhythm and intensity) and lung sounds.
- *Abdomen*: palpation, percussion, rumen motility, nasogastric intubation.
- *Head and neck*: including eyes, oral cavity, facial structures and jugular veins.
- *Rectum.*
- *Urinary tract.*
- *Reproductive tract.*
- *Mammary glands.*
- *Musculoskeletal system.*
- *Nervous system.*
- *Skin:* including ears, hooves and horns.

Multiple Choice Questions

1. What is the name for the voluntary act of forceful expiration of air through the nostrils in horses and cattle as a device to intimidate potential predators?

   a. Stridor

   b. Stertor

   c. Sneezing

   d. Snorting

2. Sudden, involuntary, noisy expiration through the nasal cavities caused reflexively by irritation of the nasal mucosae is called?

   a. Snorting

   b. Stridor

   c. Sneezing

   d. Stertor

3. Sounds caused by the presence of exudate and secretions in the airways, and oedematous bronchial mucosa are termed?

   a. Crackles

   b. Wheezes

   c. Stridor

   d. Stertor

4. Which type of dyspnoea is associated with inflammatory conditions of the upper respiratory tract, laryngitis and tracheitis?

   a. Expiratory dyspnoea

   b. Inspiratory dyspnoea

   c. Moist rales

   d. All of these

5.   **What term(s) apply to conditions with absence of breathing sounds/'silent lung' on auscultation?**

   a. Pneumothorax

   b. Hydrothorax

   c. Consolidation of lungs

   d. All of these

6.   **Which type of sounds are produced on auscultation during pulmonary emphysema?**

   a. None

   b. Extraneous

   c. Expiratory dyspnoea

   d. Inspiratory dyspnoea

7.   **What are the most pathognomic clinical signs of shock?**

   a. Tachycardia

   b. Subnormal temperature

   c. a and b

   d. None of these

8.   **What are the most accurate and sensitive methods for estimating hydration status in adult cows?**

   a. Skin tent in neck

   b. Recession of eyeballs

   c. a and b

   d. None of these

9.   **Which farm animals have true vomition phenomena?**

   a. Horses

   b. Cattle

   c. Sheep

   d. Pigs

10. **What is the shape of the abdomen in hydroperitoneum/ ascites?**

   a. Apple shaped

   b. Pappel shaped

   c. Pear shaped

   d. Drum shaped

11. **What is the condition of cattle exhibiting a papple-shaped abdomen contour?**

   a. Hofland syndrome

   b. Bloat

   c. Pregnancy

   d. Ascites

12. **The most valuable diagnostic method for the detection and localization of gas-filled viscus in the abdomen of cattle and the detection and localization of abomasal displacement is:**

   a. Ballottement

   b. Succussion

   c. Percussion and simultaneous auscultation

   d. Auscultation

13. **The most valuable diagnostic method for the detection pings indicative of intestinal tympany associated with intestinal obstruction/intestinal tympany associated with paralytic ileus in horses is:**

   a. Ballottement

   b. Percussion and simultaneous auscultation

   c. Succussion

   d. Auscultation

14. **Which clinical examination technique(s) detect floating viscera or masses in the abdominal cavity/foetus in gravid uterus?**

   a. Ballottement and auscultation

   b. Ballottement

c. Palpation

d. Auscultation

15. **Which clinical examination method is useful in detecting fluid-splashing sounds in cattle, as in grain engorgement/ left-sided abomasal displacement?**

    a. Ballottement and auscultation

    b. Ballottement

    c. Palpation

    d. Auscultation

16. **Which clinical examination method is used to detect fluid in cavities/ascites?**

    a. Ballottement

    b. Percussion

    c. Tactile percussion

    d. Percussion and simultaneous auscultation

17. **What is indicated by ping on percussion and auscultation of the left upper abdomen between the ninth and twelfth ribs and paralumbar fossa?**

    a. Left displaced abomasum

    b. Right displaced abomasum

    c. Bloat

    d. None of these

18. **Which indirect physical diagnostic test(s) are used in traumatic reticulitis?**

    a. Wither pinch test

    b. Bamboo poll test

    c. Fist test

    d. All of these

19. **In ruminants, digestive function is considered to be representative of which of these?**

    a. Ruminal motility

    b. Body temperature

    c. Peristaltic movement

    d. All of these

20. **Absence of abdominal/peristaltic sounds on auscultation in horses indicates what?**

    a. Spasmodic colic

    b. Paralytic Ileus

    c. Vagus Indigestion

    d. All of these

21. **Which of the following is a clinical examination method suitable for paranasal sinuses?**

    a. Palpation

    b. Auscultation

    c. Percussion

    d. Inspection

22. **Examination/observation of an animal from a distance is known as:**

    a. Auscultation

    b. Palpation

    c. Percussion

    d. Inspection

23. **The most suitable clinical examination method for the diagnosis of hydroperitoneum/ascites is?**

    a. Palpation

    b. Ballottement

    c. Tactile percussion

    d. Succession

24. **Cud dropping in cattle is the pathognomic clinical sign of what?**

    a. Choke

    b. Pharyngeal paralysis

    c. a and b

    d. None of these

25. **A percussion sound produced in free gas tympany in cattle and buffalo is known as:**

    a. Resonant sound

    b. Drum-like sound

    c. Dull sound

    d. Tinkling sound

26. **Which of the following is a sound produced in grain engorgement in cattle and buffalo?**

    a. Resonant sound

    b. Drum-like sound

    c. Tinkling sound

    d. Gurgling sound

27. **What shape/contour is the abdomen in ascites?**

    a. Pear shaped

    b. Apple shaped

    c. Papple shaped

    d. Drum shaped

28. **Mucous membrane colour reflects which condition of the tissues?**

    a. Oxygenation

    b. Perfusion

    c. a and b

    d. None of these

29. **Which condition(s) present with a pale mucous membrane on clinical examination?**

    a. Haemorrhagic shock

    b. Anaemia

    c. a and b

    d. Septicaemia

30. **Valvular diseases are characterised by the presence of which abnormal sound on auscultation?**

    a. Friction rub

    b. Gallop

    c. Rumbling

    d. Murmur

31. **What are the parameters used to monitor efficacy of treatment of shock?**

    a. Venous oxygen tension

    b. Blood or plasma L-lactate concentration

    c. Central venous pressure

    d. a and b

32. **What are the most useful clinical parameters for measuring the adequacy of oxygen delivery and tissue perfusion?**

    a. Venous oxygen tension

    b. Blood or plasma L-lactate concentration

    c. a and b

    d. Central venous pressure

33. **Which plasma L-lactate concentration level is indicative of anaerobic metabolism?**

    a. > 1.00 mmol/L

    b. < 2.00 mmol/L

    c. > 4.00 mmol/L

    d. > 10.00 mmol/L

34. **What colour is the mucous membrane in HCN poisoning/ histotoxic anoxia in cattle?**

   a. Bright red

   b. Cyanotic

   c. Brownish

   d. Muddy

35. **An Atropine test is used for the diagnosis of which cattle disease?**

   a. Traumatic reticulo peritonitis

   b. Left side abomasal displacement

   c. Vagus indigestion

   d. Right side abomasal displacement

36. **The mental state of an animal acting in a bizarre way and appears to be unaware of its surroundings is:**

   a. Mania

   b. Frenzy

   c. Delirium

   d. Somnolence

37. **The mental state of an animal characterized by violent activity and with little regard for surroundings is:**

   a. Mania

   b. Frenzy

   c. Somnolence

   d. Narcolepsy

38. **What is the name for episodes of uncontrolled sleep in animals?**

   a. Narcolepsy

   b. Somnolence

   c. Lassitude

   d. None of these

39. **What is the name for continuous, repetitive twitching of skeletal muscles, usually visible and palpable?**

    a. Tetany

    b. Seizures

    c. Convulsions

    d. Tremor

40. **Which disease produces tonic-clonic convulsions in goats?**

    a. Strychnine poisoning

    b. Tetanus

    c. Epilepsy

    d. All of these

41. **Which disease causes tonic convulsions in goats?**

    a. Strychnine poisoning

    b. Tetanus

    c. Epilepsy

    d. All of these

42. **Deficit of which nerve results in protrusion and deviation of the tongue, resulting in prehension of food and drinking water?**

    a. Facial nerve

    b. Glossopharyngeal nerve

    c. Hypoglossal nerve

    d. Trigeminal nerve

43. **Dysfunction in which nerve results in paralysis of the pharynx and larynx, dysphagia, regurgitation through the nostrils, abnormality of the voice and interference with respiration?**

    a. Glossopharyngeal nerve

    b. Vagus nerve

    c. a and b

    d. None of these

44. **What is the name for a sustained spasm of the neck and limb muscles resulting in dorsal and caudal extension of the head and neck with rigid extension of the limbs?**

    a. Opisthotonos

    b. Orthotonus

    c. Torticollis

    d. None of these

45. **A sustained contraction of muscles without tremor is called:**

    a. Tetany

    b. Myoclonus

    c. Tics

    d. All of these

46. **A reflex in animals showing a quick twitch of the superficial cutaneous muscle along the whole back is called:**

    a. Panniculus reflex

    b. Cutaneous trunci reflex

    c. a and b

    d. None of these

47. **An unconscious, general proprioceptive deficit causing incoordination when the animal moves is called:**

    a. Stringhalt

    b. Ataxia

    c. Hypermetria

    d. Dysmetria

48. **Paresis or paralysis with loss of voluntary movement, absence of spinal reflexes and wasting of the affected muscle (neurogenic atrophy) is caused by:**

    a. Upper motor neuron

    b. Lower motor neuron

    c. a and b

    d. None of these

49. **Neurogenic wasting of muscles is seen in lesions of:**

    a. Upper motor neuron

    b. Lower motor neuron

    c. a and b

    d. None of these

50. **Spasticity with loss of voluntary movement, increased tone of limb muscles, increased spinal reflexes is due to:**

    a. Upper motor neuron

    b. Lower motor neuron

    c. a and b

    d. None of these

51. **Brief, intermittent tetanic contraction of the skeletal muscles is known as:**

    a. Tetany

    b. Convulsions

    c. Myoclonus

    d. Tremors

52. **Defects of sacral parasympathetic outflow and the spinal sympathetic system is exhibited by signs of:**

    a. Defects of bladder sphincter control

    b. Motility of the bladder

    c. Rectum

    d. All of these

53. **Rhythmic, involuntary movement of the eyes that may occur in a horizontal, vertical, or rotary direction is known as:**

    a. Nystagmus

    b. Strabismus

    c. Blepharospasms

    d. Blepharitis

54. **Abnormal positioning of the eyeball in animals is known as:**

   a. Blepharospasms

   b. Blepharitis

   c. Nystagmus

   d. Strabismus

55. **A deficit in which nerve causes drooped ears and eyelids, drooling and retention of food in the cheek pouch?**

   a. Trigeminal nerve

   b. Facial nerve

   c. Glossopharyngeal nerve

   d. Vagus nerve

56. **Which reflex demonstrates localized twitch of the cutaneous trunci muscle elicited by tactile stimulus?**

   a. Panniculus reflex

   b. Cutaneous trunki reflex

   c. Perineal reflex

   d. a and b

57. **Which nerve is tested using the Patellar reflex?**

   a. Pudendal nerve

   b. Peroneal nerve

   c. Femoral nerve

   d. All of these

58. **Clinical examination of an animal includes:**

   a. History-taking

   b. Assessment of the animal

   c. Assessment of the environment

   d. All of these

59. **What is an indication of FAMACHA scoring in small ruminants?**

    a. Dehydration

    b. Fever

    c. Anaemia

    d. None of these

60. **What is the name for respiration demonstrating a gradual increase and then a gradual decrease in the depth?**

    a. Cheyne-Stokes

    b. Biot's

    c. Periodic breathing

    d. None of these

61. **What is the name for breathing characterized by alternating, unequal periods of hyperpnoea and apnoea?**

    a. Periodic breathing

    b. Cheyne-Stokes

    c. Biot's

    d. All of these

62. **What is the most suitable clinical diagnostic method for paranasal sinuses?**

    a. Auscultation

    b. Palpation

    c. Percussion

    d. Inspection

63. **Bran-like deposits of skin are caused by:**

    a. Urticaria

    b. Pityriasis

    c. Impetigo

    d. Pachydermia

64. **What is the word for the type of sound produced in percussion of healthy lungs?**

a. Alveolar

b. Bronchial

c. Resonant

d. Tympanic

65. **What type of sound is produced on percussion of consolidated lungs?**

a. Bronchial

b. Resonant

c. Dull

d. Tympanic

66. **What is the term for coughing up of blood?**

a. Haemoptysis

b. Hememesis

c. Epistaxis

d. Melena

67. **What is the site for recording the pulse in horses?**

a. Middle coccygeal artery

b. Facial artery

c. Femoral artery

d. Carotid artery

68. **Where should you read the pulse in goats?**

a. Carotid artery

b. Middle coccygeal artery

c. Facial artery

d. Femoral artery

69. **Where is the pulse read in bovines?**

    a. Middle coccygeal artery

    b. Facial artery

    c. Femoral artery

    d. Carotid artery

70. **A Coomb's test is used to diagnose:**

    a. Haemolytic anaemia

    b. Immune mediated haemolytic anaemia

    c. Haemorrhagic anaemia

    d. All of these

71. **Haemorrhage of which part of the gastrointestinal tract makes the faeces tarry in appearance?**

    a. Stomach

    b. Large Intestine

    c. Colon

    d. Caecum

72. **What term is used for haemorrhage in the lower colon and rectum causing the voiding of clots of whole blood?**

    a. Melena

    b. Haematochezia

    c. a and b

    d. None of these

73. **What colour are the faeces in obstructive jaundice?**

    a. Tar coloured

    b. Clay coloured

    c. Brown

    d. Yellow

74. **Which disease does not produce rigor mortis?**

a. Strangles

b. Enterotoxaemia

c. Anthrax

d. Glanders

75. **What is a diagnostic marker for complete extrahepatic biliary obstruction?**

a. Absence of urobilinogen

b. Presence of urobilinogen

c. Presence of urine bilirubin

d. None of these

76. **What are the clinico-pathological findings in intravascular haemolysis jaundice?**

a. Hemoglobinemia

b. Haemoglobinuria

c. Jaundice

d. All of these

77. **Which characteristic clinico-pathological finding is not present in extravascular haemolysis jaundice?**

a. Hemoglobinemia

b. Haemoglobinuria

c. a and b

d. None of these

78. **The best indicator of the hydration status in dairy calves is:**

a. Recession of eyeball into the orbit

b. Capillary refill time

c. Skin tent

d. All of these

79. **What type of sound is heard in atrioventricular valvular insufficiency?**

   a. Systolic murmurs

   b. Diastolic murmurs

   c. Continuous murmurs

   d. None of these

80. **What type of sound is heard in pulmonic or aortic valvular insufficiency?**

   a. Systolic murmurs

   b. Diastolic murmurs

   c. Continuous murmurs

   d. None of these

81. **What type of sound is heard in abnormal orifices in the heart or ductus arteriosus?**

   a. Systolic murmurs

   b. Diastolic murmurs

   c. Continuous murmurs

   d. None of these

82. **Which condition has the clinical sign of jugular engorgement in cows?**

   a. Right-side congestive heart failure

   b. Left-side congestive heart failure

   c. a and b

   d. None of these

83. **Which type of dyspnoea is usually associated with diffuse or advanced obstructive lower airway disease?**

   a. Expiratory dyspnoea

   b. Inspiratory dyspnoea

   c. Open-mouth breathing

   d. Coughing

84. **Which type of dyspnoea is usually associated with diffuse or advanced obstructive upper airway/extra-thoracic airway diseases?**

a. Expiratory dyspnoea

b. Coughing

c. Inspiratory dyspnoea

d. Open-mouth breathing

85. **Which disease causes arrhythmias and conduction disturbances?**

a. Endocarditis

b. Myocarditis

c. Pericarditis

d. All of these

86. **What type of murmurs are associated with stenosis of the outflow valves or insufficiency of the atrioventricular valves?**

a. Systolic murmurs

b. Diastolic murmurs

c. Continuous murmurs

d. Hemic murmurs

87. **Which murmurs are associated with insufficiency of the outflow valves or stenosis of the atrioventricular valves?**

a. Systolic murmurs

b. Diastolic murmurs

c. Continuous murmurs

d. Hemic murmurs

88. **Dribbling of urine from the umbilicus in foals is known as:**

a. Urolithiasis

b. Nephroliths

c. Pervious urachus

d. All of these

89. **The commonest site for uroliths in rams and lodging uroliths in bucks is:**

    a. Ischial arch

    b. Sigmoid flexure

    c. Urethral process

    d. b and c

90. **A major clinical manifestation of ectopic ureters at birth in foals is known as:**

    a. Periuria

    b. Dysuria

    c. Anuria

    d. Urinary incontinence

91. **An increase in the volume of urine produced over a 24-hour period is called:**

    a. Pollakiuria

    b. Periuria

    c. Polyuria

    d. All of these

92. **An increase in frequency of urination usually accompanied by a decreased volume of urine is known as:**

    a. Pollakiuria

    b. Periuria

    c. Polyuria

    d. All of these

93. **What is the odour of urine in acute cystitis?**

    a. Sweet

    b. Sour

    c. Strong ammoniacal

    d. None of these

94. **Which test is used to differentiate prerenal, renal, or postrenal azotaemia?**

    a. Urine pH

    b. Urine creatinine

    c. Urine protein

    d. Specific gravity of urine

95. **What is the normal pulse rate per minute in cattle?**

    a. 42–60

    b. 33–41

    c. 60–70

    d. 120–130

96. **What is the normal pulse rate per minute in horses?**

    a. 42–60

    b. 33–41

    c. 60–70

    d. 120–130

97. **What is the normal pulse rate per minute in sheep?**

    a. 60–70

    b. 42–62

    c. 100–120

    d. 33–41

98. **Voiding small quantities of stool with mucus is characteristic of:**

    a. Small bowel diarrhoea

    b. Large bowel diarrhoea

    c. a and b

    d. None of these

99. **What is the aetiology of goose-stepping gait in pigs?**

    a. Vitamin A

    b. Vitamin B$_1$

c. Vitamin B_5

d. Vitamin B_3

100. **Wheal-like cutaneous eruptions of the skin due to hypersensitivity are known as:**

   a. Erythema

   b. Urticaria

   c. Blister

   d. Boil

101. **What is the effect of *Lantana camara* plant toxicity in animals?**

   a. Photosensitization

   b. Hepatotoxicity

   c. Nephrotoxicity

   d. a and b

102. **A depressive state of animal behaviour is known as:**

   a. Anxiety

   b. Frenzy

   c. Mania

   d. Somnolence

103. **The most potent cardiac bio-marker in cattle is:**

   a. ALT

   b. CPK

   c. Troponin-I

   d. Amylase

104. **Murmurs on auscultation without valvular lesions are associated with:**

   a. AV stenosis

   b. Anaemia

   c. Hypoproteinaemia

   d. b and c

105. **Which if these is a major cause of loss in neonatal pigs?**

   a. Hypothermia from heat loss

   b. Hypothermia/hypoglycaemia from starvation

   c. Colibacillosis

   d. a and b

106. **Which blood test is used to measure tissue oxygen transport and cellular metabolism?**

   a. Blood lactate

   b. Blood oxygen

   c. Blood carbon dioxide

   d. All of these

107. **Which is the most sensitive indicator of muscle damage?**

   a. Creatinine kinase

   b. Alkaline phosphatase

   c. a and b

   d. None of these

108. **What is the odour of the urine in acute cystitis?**

   a. Ammoniacal

   b. Sweet

   c. Aromatic

   d. No change

109. **Plant toxicity in ruminants showing gangrenous extremities and hyperthermia in cattle is:**

   a. Ergot

   b. Nux Vomica

   c. Reserpine

   d. Gossypol

110. **What might be a tentative diagnosis for a dead animal with half-chewed food in its mouth?**

   a. Electrocution

   b. Lightning stroke

   c. a and b

   d. None of these

111. **Guttural pouch empyema in horses occurs due to which infection?**

   a. Strangles

   b. Anthrax

   c. Glanders

   d. Botulism

112. **Which disease of horses produces nodules, ulcers, scar formation and a debilitated condition?**

   a. Strangles

   b. Anthrax

   c. Glanders

   d. Botulism

113. **Which disease of swine demonstrates haemorrhages, purplish skin discoloration of the ears, lower abdomen and legs?**

   a. Classical swine fever

   b. African swine fever

   c. a and b

   d. None of these

114. **Abducted elbows and careful gait in cattle indicate:**

   a. Pleurisy

   b. Pericarditis

   c. TRP

   d. All of these

115. **Auscultation in the effusive stage of traumatic pericarditis has what type of sound?**

    a. Pericardial friction rub

    b. Muffled heart sound

    c. Murmurs

    d. None of these

116. **An increase in body temperature due to pyrogens and regardless of external temperature indicates:**

    a. Fever

    b. Hyperthermia

    c. Heat stroke

    d. All of these

117. **A sensation of breathlessness in a recumbent position, relieved by sitting or standing is known as:**

    a. Orthopnoea

    b. Dyspnoea

    c. Apnoea

    d. Polypnoea

118. **What are the characteristics of large bowel diarrhoea?**

    a. Small faecal volume

    b. Tenesmus

    c. Presence of mucus

    d. All of these

119. **What are the characteristics of small bowel diarrhoea?**

    a. Haematochezia

    b. Presence of mucus

    c. Voluminous stool

    d. Tenesmus

120. **Electrolyte imbalance with clinical signs resembling botulism with flaccid paralysis of the tongue and masticatory muscles and the head resting on the ground indicates:**

   a. Hypocalcaemia

   b. Hypomagnesemia

   c. Hypokalaemia

   d. Hyperkalaemia

121. **Post parturient hyperesthesia, tetany, tachycardia and convulsions in cows beyond the first stage of parturient paresis is known as:**

   a. Hypomagnesemia

   b. Hypophosphatemia

   c. Ketosis

   d. Metritis

122. **What is the name of the enzyme associated with degenerative myopathy?**

   a. CK

   b. ALT

   c. AST

   d. BUN

123. **Which disorder in ewes in the last month of pregnancy exhibits encephalopathy with blindness, muscle tremors, convulsions and metabolic acidosis?**

   a. Ketosis

   b. Pregnancy toxaemia

   c. Milk fever

   d. Hypomagnesemia

124. **Which is the most reliable and inexpensive cowside test for detecting subclinical mastitis?**

   a. Somatic cell count

   b. Electric conductivity

c. California mastitis test

d. All of these

125. **An indirect measure of the prevalence of mastitis within a dairy herd is:**

a. Bulk tank milk somatic cell counts

b. Bulk tank bacterial culture

c. Bulk tank electric conductivity

d. All of these

126. **The NAGase activity test is used in the diagnosis of:**

a. Enteritis

b. Chronic kidney failure

c. Mastitis

d. Brucellosis

127. **Which test is used to measure actual injury to the udder rather than the cow's response to the damage?**

a. Electrical conductivity

b. Somatic cell count

c. NAGase activity

d. All of these

128. **Which test is used to measure a cow's response to udder damage rather than actual injury to the udder?**

a. Somatic cell count

b. NAGase activity

c. a and b

d. None of these

129. **What is the name for flat-topped, steep-walled, solid elevations of the skin arising from histamine release?**

a. Papules

b. Nodules

c. Wheals

d. Vesicles

130. **What is the name of the photosensitizing agent which accumulates in plasma in impaired hepatobiliary excretion in cattle?**

a. Phylloerythrin

b. Chlorophyll

c. a and b

d. None of these

131. **Which type of photosensitivity is due to aberrant pigment metabolism (photosensitizing porphyrin) arising from defective functions of enzymes involved in heme synthesis?**

a. Type I

b. Type II

c. Type III

d. Type IV

132. **In horses, a cutaneous manifestation of acute-onset hypersensitivity, with haired, dome-shaped wheals in horses is called a:**

a. Urticaria

b. Hive

c. a and b

d. None of these

133. **What is the name for deficient pigmentation in hair or wool fibre?**

a. Achromotrichia

b. Leukoderma

c. Vitiligo

d. All of these

134. **What is the name for a congenital lack of melatonin pigment in the skin, hair and other normally pigmented tissues?**

    a. Albinism

    b. Leukoderma

    c. Vitiligo

    d. Leucotrichia

135. **What is the name for a soft, painless, fluctuating subcutaneous swelling, crepitant to the touch but without external skin lesions?**

    a. Gas gangrene

    b. Subcutaneous emphysema

    c. Oedema

    d. None of these

136. **Moist and oozy skin with swelling, discolouration, cold to the touch and with demarcation from healthy skin is known as:**

    a. Abscess

    b. Gangrene

    c. Haematoma

    d. Emphysema

137. **Which type of gangrene is caused by arterial occlusions resulting in tissue ischemia?**

    a. Dry gangrene

    b. Wet gangrene

    c. Gas gangrene

    d. None of these

138. **What is the name for transient, localized subcutaneous oedema resulting from an allergic reaction in cattle?**

    a. Anasarca

    b. Angioedema

    c. Purpura haemorrhagica

    d. None of these

139. **Mastitis metritis dysagalactia is common in:**

    a. Sows

    b. Mares

    c. Cows

    d. Does

140. **Failure of provisional calcification of the osteoid, plus failure of mineralization of the cartilaginous matrix of developing bone, is known as:**

    a. Osteodystrophia fibrosa

    b. Osteomalacia

    c. Rickets

    d. Osteoporosis

141. **What condition afflicts horses with a diet high in bran, showing swelling of the mandibles, maxillae and frontal bones ('bighead' syndrome)?**

    a. Osteodystrophia fibrosa

    b. Osteomalacia

    c. Rickets

    d. Osteoporosis

142. **Which condition demonstrates long bones without any distortion in shape but demineralization and softening, leading to spontaneous fracture?**

    a. Osteodystrophia fibrosa

    b. Osteomalacia

    c. Rickets

    d. Osteoporosis

143. **Inflammation of any adipose tissue is known as?**

    a. Steatitis

    b. Folliculitis

    c. Yellow fat disease

    d. a and c

144. **Silage feeding is associated with which disease in ruminants?**

    a. Leptospirosis

    b. Cerebrocortical necrosis

    c. Salmonellosis

    d. Listeriosis

145. **The gold standard test for subclinical ketosis is:**

    a. BHB measurement

    b. NEFA estimation

    c. a and b

    d. Glucose

146. **Which condition is associated with high plasma BHB concentrations?**

    a. Ketosis

    b. Left displacement of abomasum

    c. Reduced fertility

    d. All of these

147. **Toxicity in cattle causing mottled, chalky, pitted and stained enamel and excessive wear on the teeth is known as:**

    a. Fluoride oxicity

    b. Selenium toxicity

    c. Arsenic toxicity

    d. Molybdenum

148. **The most accurate test for the diagnosis of ketosis in cattle is:**

    a. BHB measurement

    b. NEFA estimation

    c. a and b

    d. None of these

149. **Metabolic tests to monitor energy balance in prepartum dairy cows are known as:**

   a. Plasma/serum NEFA

   b. Plasma/serum BHB

   c. Plasma/serum glucose

   d. All of these

150. **Which disorder is caused due to deficiency of copper in calves?**

   a. Peat scours

   b. Teart

   c. Falling disease

   d. All of these

151. **What is the aetiology of hepatosis dietetica in pigs?**

   a. Deficiency of copper

   b. Excess of molybdenum

   c. Deficiency of Vita-E and Se

   d. High-energy diet

152. **White liver disease in sheep is caused by:**

   a. Co deficiency

   b. Cu deficiency

   c. Se deficiency

   d. Mn deficiency

153. **Dorsal side bending of the spinal column in animals is called:**

   a. Lordosis

   b. Kyphosis

   c. Scoliosis

   d. Torticollis

154. **Ventral side bending of the spinal column in animals is called:**

    a. Lordosis

    b. Kyphosis

    c. Scoliosis

    d. Torticollis

155. **Lateral side bending of the spinal column in animals is known as:**

    a. Lordosis

    b. Kyphosis

    c. Scoliosis

    d. Torticollis

156. **An involuntary unilateral contraction of the neck muscles causing torsion (twisting) of the neck is referred to as:**

    a. Kyphosis

    b. Scoliosis

    c. Lordosis

    d. Torticollis

157. **The major cause of mortality in neonatal piglets is:**

    a. Hypoglycaemia

    b. Hypothermia

    c. a and b

    d. None of these

158. **Which neonates require a steady supply of milk as energy?**

    a. Piglets

    b. Calves

    c. Foals

    d. None of these

159. **What is the name for a disease in horses causing forceful, double efforts for expiration, flared nostrils, heave line and wheezing during expiration?**

   a. Chronic obstructive pulmonary disease

   b. Broken wind

   c. Heaves

   d. All of these

160. **Which of the following is a viral disease of cattle demonstrating shifting lameness and pyrexia?**

   a. Foot and mouth disease

   b. Foot rot

   c. Ephemeral disease

   d. Joint ill

161. **Name the highly contagious disease in ruminants causing panting, permanent loss of milk production, lack of heat tolerance and overgrowth of hairs?**

   a. Bovine viral diarrhoea

   b. Vesicular stomatitis

   c. Aphthous fever

   d. Vesicular exanthema

162. **Which disease in goats exhibits as pyrexia, nasal discharge, necrotic greyish mouth lesions and diarrhoea?**

   a. Contagious ecthyma

   b. Peste des petits

   c. Vesicular stomatitis

   d. Foot and mouth disease

163. **Sudden death in cows without premonitory signs, with bloody discharge from the mouth, nostrils and anus is caused by:**

   a. Black quarter

   b. Anthrax

c. Lightning stroke

d. HCN poisoning

164. **Abortion storm in cows in the third trimester and orchitis and epididymitis in bulls are symptoms of:**

    a. Trichomoniasis

    b. Vibriosis

    c. Leptospirosis

    d. Brucellosis

165. **The Rose Bengal test is used in the diagnosis of:**

    a. Brucellosis

    b. Trichomoniasis

    c. Vibriosis

    d. Listeriosis

166. **Which swine disease has clinical signs of diamond- or rhomboid-shaped urticarial skin lesions?**

    a. Swine erysipelas

    b. African swine disease

    c. Classical swine disease

    d. None of these

167. **Localised chronic, progressive, granulomatous abscesses involving the mandible or maxilla, or other bony tissues of the head, result from:**

    a. Actinomycosis

    b. Wooden tongue

    c. Osteodystrophy fibosa

    d. All of these

168. **What is the name for a disease in cattle with peripheral (centripetal) corneal opacity as an important clinical sign?**

    a. Malignant catarrhal fever

    b. Bovine viral diarrhoea

    c. Rinderpest

    d. Mucosal disease

169. **Which disease shows a severe immunosuppressive effect, thrombocytopenia, haemorrhagic enteritis, pneumonia, abortions, infertility and/or embryonic death?**

    a. BVD

    b. MCF

    c. FMD

    d. RP

170. **Pathognomic post-mortem lesions in goats, showing zebra markings in the intestine, suggest:**

    a. PPR

    b. RP

    c. Contagious ecthyma

    d. Bluetongue

171. **Which disease has characteristic post-mortem lesions, and a 'turkey-egg' appearance to the kidneys?**

    a. Classical swine fever

    b. Bovine viral diarrhoea

    c. Mucosal disease

    d. African horse sickness

172. **Tick-borne encephalitis showing fine muscular tremors, nervous nibbling, ataxia, weakness and collapse is known as:**

    a. Scrapie

    b. Louping ill

    c. Visna

    d. Maedi

173. **Which disease has characteristic pipe-stem stools in cattle?**

    a. *Babesia bovis*

    b. *Babesia divergens*

    c. a and b

    d. None of these

174. **Which type of clinical signs are exhibited by equine herpes virus-1?**

    a. Respiratory

    b. Abortion

    c. Neurological

    d. All of these

175. **Horses showing ataxia or wobbly gait, urine retention/dribbling, bladder atony and recumbency, often preceded by fever and/or respiratory signs, are likely to be suffering from:**

    a. Equine herpes virus-1

    b. Equine infectious anaemia

    c. African horse sickness

    d. None of these

176. **What is another name for African horse sickness in foals?**

    a. Dunkop

    b. Dikkop

    c. a and b

    d. None of these

177. **What is the name for the sub-acute form of African horse sickness in foals?**

    a. Dunkop

    b. Dikkop

    c. a and b

    d. None of these

178. **Which disease is associated with suppurative bursitis, recognized as fistulous withers or poll evil in horses?**

    a. *Brucella spp.*

    b. *Streptococcus spp.*

c. *Staphylococcus spp.*

d. *Clostridium spp.*

179. **Which test is used to monitor brucellosis in a dairy herd?**

   a. Milk ring

   b. Slide agglutination

   c. White side

   d. None of these

180. **Glasser's disease is characterized by which clinical sign in pigs?**

   a. Fibrinous polyseositis

   b. Polyarthritis

   c. Bronchopneumonia

   d. All of these

181. **Diamond skin disease of pigs, showing diffuse erythema, septicaemia and/or arthritis is known as:**

   a. Swine erysipelas

   b. *Salmonella choleraesuis*

   c. Classical swine fever

   d. *Streptococcus suis*

182. **Heamagalactia is a clinical sign of which disease in cows?**

   a. Actinobacillosis

   b. Anthrax

   c. Leptospirosis

   d. All of these

183. **Which serological test is used for screening at the herd level for leptospirosis in cows?**

   a. MAT

   b. ELISA

   c. CFT

   d. All of these

184. **What is the correct titre for a microagglutination test (MAT) considered for evidence of leptospirosis in cattle?**

    a. ≥ 1600

    b. ≥ 800

    c. ≥ 400

    d. ≥ 200

185. **Which disease of ruminants is associated with eating poor quality silage with a pH > 5–5.5?**

    a. Listeriosis

    b. Leptospirosis

    c. Botulism

    d. None of these

186. **In ruminants, which disease causes localized asymmetric ascending infection resulting in meningoencephalitis?**

    a. Botulism

    b. Pregnancy toxaemia

    c. Listeriosis

    d. Polioencephalomalacia

187. **'Hard udder' syndrome in goats is characterized by a firm, swollen mammary gland and agalactia at the time of parturition. What is the official name for this condition?**

    a. *Mycoplasma*

    b. Caprine arthritis encephalitis disease

    c. Maedi-visna

    d. None of these

188. **Which disease in small ruminants is caused by lentivirus?**

    a. Ovine progressive pneumonia

    b. Caprine arthritis and encephalitis

    c. a and b

    d. None of these

189. The larval stage of the parasite that inhabits the nasal passages and sinuses of sheep and goats is called:

    a. *Oestrus ovis*

    b. *Trichuris vulpis*

    c. *Haemonchus* spp.

    d. *Bunostomum* spp.

190. Which organ is inhabited by the larval stage of the parasite *Oestrus ovis* in sheep and goats?

    a. Skin

    b. Small intestine

    c. Caecum

    d. Nasal passages

191. Which of these is a viral disease in goats characterized by fever, necrotic stomatitis, conjunctivitis, gastroenteritis, pneumonia and sometimes death?

    a. Contagious caprine pleuropneumonia

    b. Contagious ecthyma

    c. Heartwater

    d. Peste des petits ruminants

192. Which disease is most commonly seen during the first weeks of life and in immunocompromised neonates?

    a. Colisepticemia

    b. Joint ill

    c. Meningitis

    d. All of these

193. Which chronic, contagious granulomatous enteritis is characterized in cattle by progressive weight loss, debilitation and eventually death?

    a. Paratuberculosis

    b. Tuberculosis

c. Bovine viral diarrhoea

d. All of these

194. **Transient loss of consciousness due to ischemia or lower supply of oxygen to the brain is known as:**

a. Syncope

b. Coma

c. Epilepsy

d. None of these

195. **What is indicated by an ECG with no P waves discernible but the baseline having multiple waveforms (F waves)?**

a. Atrial fibrillation

b. Ventricular tachycardia

c. AV block

d. Sinus arrhythmia

196. **AV block with a gradual increase in the PQ interval up to the point of the blocked conduction is termed:**

a. Mobitz type 1

b. First degree AV block

c. Third degree AV block

d. Mobitz type II

197. **What is indicated by an ECG showing a slow and independent ventricular rate characterized by QRS complexes that are completely dissociated from the faster P waves?**

a. Complete heart block

b. Wandering pacemaker

c. Atrial standstill

d. None of these

198. **What is the term for an arterial pulse of large amplitude with high systolic and low diastolic blood pressure?**

    a. Thready pulse

    b. Bounding pulse

    c. Water hammer pulse

    d. None of these

199. **Cranial nerve dysfunction with bilateral drooping of the ear, ptosis of the upper eyelid, drooping of the lips and pulling of the philtrum to the unaffected side relates to which nerve?**

    a. Oculomotor

    b. Glossopharyngeal

    c. Facial

    d. Trigeminal

Answers

1.	d	31.	d	61.	c	91.	c
2.	c	32.	c	62.	c	92.	a
3.	a	33.	c	63.	b	93.	c
4.	b	34.	a	64.	c	94.	d
5.	d	35.	c	65.	c	95.	a
6.	c	36.	a	66.	a	96.	b
7.	c	37.	b	67.	b	97.	a
8.	c	38.	a	68.	d	98.	b
9.	d	39.	d	69.	a	99.	c
10.	d	40.	c	70.	b	100.	b
11.	a	41.	b	71.	a	101.	d
12.	c	42.	c	72.	b	102.	d
13.	b	43.	c	73.	c	103.	c
14.	b	44.	a	74.	c	104.	d
15.	a	45.	a	75.	a	105.	d
16.	c	46.	c	76.	d	106.	a
17.	a	47.	b	77.	d	107.	a
18.	d	48.	b	78.	a	108.	a
19.	a	49.	b	79.	a	109.	a
20.	b	50.	a	80.	b	110.	c
21.	c	51.	c	81.	c	111.	a
22.	d	52.	d	82.	a	112.	c
23.	c	53.	a	83.	a	113.	c
24.	c	54.	d	84.	c	114.	d
25.	b	55.	b	85.	b	115.	b
26.	d	56.	d	86.	a	116.	a
27.	b	57.	c	87.	b	117.	a
28.	c	58.	d	88.	c	118.	d
29.	c	59.	c	89.	c	119.	c
30.	d	60.	a	90.	b	120.	c

(Continued)

121.	a	141.	a	161.	c	181.	a
122.	a	142.	b	162.	b	182.	c
123.	b	143.	d	163.	b	183.	a
124.	c	144.	d	164.	d	184.	b
125.	a	145.	a	165.	a	185.	a
126.	c	146.	d	166.	a	186.	c
127.	a	147.	a	167.	a	187.	b
128.	c	148.	a	168.	a	188.	c
129.	c	149.	a	169.	a	189.	a
130.	a	150.	d	170.	a	190.	d
131.	b	151.	c	171.	a	191.	d
132.	c	152.	a	172.	b	192.	d
133.	a	153.	b	173.	c	193.	a
134.	a	154.	a	174.	d	194.	a
135.	b	155.	c	175.	a	195.	a
136.	b	156.	d	176.	a	196.	a
137.	a	157.	c	177.	b	197.	a
138.	b	158.	a	178.	a	198.	c
139.	a	159.	d	179.	a	199.	c
140.	c	160.	c	180.	d		

3 Electrolyte Balance and Fluid Therapy

S. Yogeshpriya, L. Sowmiya, S. Sivaraman and D. Sumathi

Introduction

Fluid therapy is the administration of fluids to a patient as a treatment or preventative measure. It can be administered via intravenous, intraperitoneal, subcutaneous and oral routes. Fluid therapy in animals is often difficult. The cost and the time it takes to properly restrain a cow, administer the volume needed and monitor the animal makes us often reluctant to correct fluid imbalances properly in adult cattle. It is necessary to discuss fluid therapy of mature cattle separately from fluid therapy of calves because the metabolic abnormalities commonly seen in mature cattle are quite different from those of calves and other species. The underlying cause needs to be identified and corrected, but fluid therapy is often a key factor in the recovery process. The type of fluid, the volume and the route the fluids are to be given will help to correct circulatory collapse, electrolyte imbalances and base deficits.

Certain emergency conditions of adult cattle cause different degrees of fluid and electrolyte deficits and changes in the animal's acid-base status. Often, it is not practical to perform laboratory analysis when working as a field vet. It would mean taking a blood sample, driving back to the surgery to analyse it and then back to the farm to administer the right fluids. What we do know is that in adult cattle, conditions such as grain overload and choke cause an acidotic state. We also know that gastrointestinal catastrophes such as abomasal volvulus and caecal or abomasal torsion result in a metabolic alkalosis. Circulatory collapse is often a result of endotoxaemia caused by per acute Gram-negative bacterial infections, such as *Escherichia coli* mastitis, severe endometritis and septic peritonitis. In these above-mentioned scenarios, correction of dehydration will often restore renal function sufficiently that electrolyte and acid-based imbalances will then self-correct.

© CAB International 2024. *Key Questions in Clinical Farm Animal Medicine Volume 1: Principles of Disease Examination, Diagnosis and Management* (ed. T. Rana)
DOI: 10.1079/9781800624788.0003

When addressing hydration status, body weight and rumen fill can be misleading, as can skin tent time and eyeball recession – for example, animals in poor body condition will have skin that tents and retracted eyeballs, regardless of their hydration status. Clinical signs vary between the various degrees of dehydration in adult ruminants.

Multiple Choice Questions

1. **What is the most clinical sign of decreased plasma osmotic pressure?**

   a. Localized oedema

   b. Generalized oedema

   c. Subcutaneous oedema

   d. Ascites

2. **The secondary response to continued negative water balance is a reduction in the fluid content of the blood causing a:**

   a. Reduction in circulating blood volume

   b. Increase in concentration of blood

   c. Increase in circulating blood volume

   d. a and b

3. **The most accurate and sensitive method to assess hydration status is:**

   a. Eye recession

   b. Skin tent duration

   c. a and b

   d. None of these

4. **The rapid ingestion of a large quantity of water by animals with increased serum sodium concentration leads to:**

   a. Intravascular haemolysis

   b. Haemoglobinuria

   c. Hemoglobinemia

   d. Cerebral oedema

5. **The ion responsible for the maintenance of osmotic pressure of extracellular fluid is:**

   a. Chloride

   b. Sodium

    c. Magnesium

    d. Calcium

6. **Polyurea and polydipsia occur in cattle with a dietary deficiency of:**

    a. Magnesium

    b. Sodium chloride

    c. Potassium

    d. Potassium chloride

7. **The treatment of ketosis in lactating dairy cows with multiple dosages of isoflupredone, a glucocorticoid with some mineralocorticoid activity, can cause:**

    a. Hyperkalaemia

    b. Hypokalaemia

    c. Hypocalcaemia

    d. Hypomagnesemia

8. **The method of choice for treating lactating dairy cattle with hypokalaemia is administration of potassium:**

    a. Orally

    b. Intravenously

    c. a and b

    d. Subcutaneously

9. **The preferred forms of calcium for intravenous administration are:**

    a. Calcium gluconate and calcium chloride

    b. Calcium borogluconate and calcium gluconate

    c. Calcium chloride and calcium propionate

    d. Calcium borogluconate and calcium chloride

10. **The dose of Calcium borogluconate for an adult lactating cow with periparturient hypocalcaemia is**

   a. 500 ml of 23% Calcium borogluconate

   b. 500 ml of 23% Calcium chloride

   c. 500 ml of 23% Calcium gluconate

   d. 500 ml of 23% Calcium propionate

11. **The monobasic monophosphate form of sodium phosphate is used for treating:**

   a. Hypokalaemia

   b. Hypophosphatemia

   c. Hypernatremia

   d. Hyponatremia

12. **Accumulation of oedematous transudate in subcutaneous tissues is known as:**

   a. Anasarca

   b. Ascites

   c. Hydrothorax

   d. Hydropericardium

13. **The following are unfavourable responses during intravenous fluid therapy, except:**

   a. Dyspnoea

   b. Urination within 30 to 60 minutes

   c. Failure to urinate

   d. Tetany

14. **Dehydrated mammals in hot environments can save water by reducing the rate of:**

   a. Panting

   b. Sweating

   c. a and b

   d. Respiration

15.   **In dehydration, fluid drains primarily from:**

a. Intracellular and interstitial fluid spaces

b. Interstitial and extracellular fluid spaces

c. Extracellular fluid spaces

d. Circulation

16.   **Haemoconcentration causes an increase in the viscosity of blood which impedes blood flow and causes:**

a. Systemic circulation failure

b. Peripheral circulatory failure

c. Diapedesis

d. Bleeding

17.   **Which of these is a significant avenue of evaporative heat loss in goats when exposed to temperatures of above 40 °C?**

a. Panting

b. Tachypnoea

c. Bradycardia

d. Sweating

18.   **In calves with acute diarrhoea and normal water intake, the organ which compensates very effectively for faecal water loss and plasma volume maintenance is:**

a. Urethra

b. Urinary bladder

c. Kidney

d. Ureter

19.   **Which of the following compensatory measures taken by the body to cope with dehydration is correct?**

i.   Dry faeces

ii. Decreased urine output

iii. Increased sweat

iv. Decreased sweat

a. All are correct

b. i, ii, iv correct, iii incorrect

c. i, ii correct, iii, iv incorrect

d. i, iii correct, ii, iv incorrect

20. **Simple deprivation of water leads to:**

a. Hypertonic dehydration

b. Hypotonic dehydration

c. Isotonic dehydration

d. Urolithiasis

21. **Enterotoxigenic colibacillosis leads to:**

a. Hypertonic dehydration

b. Hypotonic dehydration

c. Isotonic dehydration

d. Urolithiasis

22. **Copious sweating, nephrosis and simple enteritis leads to:**

a. Hypertonic dehydration

b. Hypotonic dehydration

c. Isotonic dehydration

d. Urolithiasis

23. **Consider the following statements: which of them is true?**

i. Metabolic alkalosis and hypokalaemia in cattle is accompanied by muscular weakness and paradoxical aciduria

ii. Hypokalaemia caused by lowering the resting membrane potential of membranes results in decreased excitability of neuromuscular tissue

iii. Calves with neonatal diarrhoea can have marked depletion of body potassium stores

iv. Hypokalaemia causes prolonged recumbency, inability to hold up the head and muscle tremors

a. i true

b. i and ii true

c. i, ii and iii true

d. All are true

24. **A large amount of chloride is secreted in what by the mucosal cells in exchange for bicarbonate, which moves into plasma?**

a. Omasum

b. Abomasum

c. Rumen

d. Reticulum

25. **Intravenous therapy for hypokalaemia involves administration of isotonic solution of 1.15% KCl which should be administered at less than:**

a. 3.2 ml/kg/hr

b. 2.2 ml/kg/hr

c. 1.2 ml/kg/hr

d. 4.2 ml/kg/hr

26. **Intravenous administration of higher rates of potassium causes:**

a. Arrhythmia

b. Ventricular premature complex

c. Ventricular fibrillation

d. All of these

27. **The potassium concentration in the rumen fluid of cattle is:**

a. 24 to 85 mmol/L

b. 24 to 85 meq/L

c. 24 to 85 mmol/ml

d. 24 to 85 meq/ml

28. **For a 600 kg dairy cow, the current recommendation for treatment of hypokalaemia is to administer food grade potassium chloride at the dose rate of:**

    a. 120 g twice a day

    b. 240 g twice a day

    c. 120 g once a day

    d. 420 g once a day

29. **The effect of hyperkalaemia on the ECG is exacerbated by the presence of what, which is common in neonatal calves with diarrhoea?**

    a. Hypocalcaemia

    b. Hyponatraemia

    c. Hypercalcaemia

    d. Hypochloraemia

30. **Intravenous administration of 500 ml of 23% calcium boro-gluconate provides calcium of about:**

    a. 10.7 g

    b. 15.7 g

    c. 1.07 g

    d. 5.35 g

31. **The gradual decrease in the depth of respiration in renal and cardiac disease is known as:**

    a. Kausmal's respiration

    b. Cheyne's stoke respiration

    c. Eupnoea

    d. Biot's respiration

32. **Hypoalbuminaemia can result from:**

    a. Blood sucking parasites

    b. Bleeding into third spaces such as the peritoneal and pleural cavities

c. Decreased production of protein or decreased intake

d. All of these

33.   **Plasma proteins are synthesized from:**

a. Liver

b. Spleen

c. Bone marrow

d. None of these

34.   **Increased hydrostatic pressure can be caused by:**

a. Chronic blood loss

b. Symmetric ventral and pulmonary oedema

c. Chronic liver disease

d. Toxic damage to vascular epithelium

35.   **Oncotic pressure of plasma is decreased by:**

a. Protein-losing enteropathy

b. Local oedema

c. Compressive lesions

d. Allergic oedema

36.   **Total body water and electrolytes are maintained at a homeostatic level by the buffering system of:**

a. Blood

b. Lungs

c. Kidney

d. All of these

37.   **Acidosis in grain overload in cattle may be fatal within:**

a. 4 days

b. 24–48 hours

c. 1 week

d. 12 hours

38. **What is common in new born animals with metabolic acidosis?**

   a. They stand unsteadily

   b. Lack of suckling reflex

   c. Lack of palpebral reflex

   d. All of these

39. **The severity of water loss is indicated by:**

   a. Packed cell volume

   b. Total serum protein

   c. a and b

   d. Mental depression

40. **Intensive fluid therapy is necessary if the PCV value goes above:**

   a. 30

   b. 40

   c. 50

   d. 60

41. **The normal total serum protein concentration is:**

   a. 2–4 g/dl

   b. 6–7.5 g/dl

   c. 8–10 g/dl

   d. 12 g/dl

42. **The metabolic breakdown constituents that can be used to assess the degree of dehydration and distinguish between prerenal, renal and postrenal uraemia are:**

   a. Urea and creatinine

   b. Urea and citrulline

   c. Ammonia and creatinine

   d. Urea and ammonia

43. **Plasma urea and creatinine concentrations vary directly in relation to the intake of which two things, respectively, in healthy animals?**

   a. Protein, muscle mass

   b. Muscle mass, protein

   c. Protein, water

   d. Water, protein

44. **Hypertonic saline solution is given intravenously over a period of 4 to 5 minutes at the rate of:**

   a. 2 to 3ml/kg

   b. 4 to 5 ml/kg

   c. 90 to 100 ml/kg

   d. 10 to15 ml/kg

45. **Which type of respiration is characterized by alternating periods of hyperpnoea and apnoea, seen in meningitis?**

   a. Kausmal's respiration

   b. Cheyne's stoke respiration

   c. Eupnoea

   d. Biot's respiration

46. **Which test is used for the estimation of calcium in the urine in hypocalcaemia?**

   a. Sulkowich test

   b. Xylidil test

   c. Hoti's test

   d. Cmt

47. **'Air hunger' is a type of respiration which is forceful and regular, but expiration is unaffected – seen in uraemia and diabetic ketoacidosis. It is also known as:**

   a. Kausmal's respiration

   b. Cheyne's stoke respiration

c. Eupnoea

d. Biot's respiration

48. **The conditions that are accompanied by respiratory acidosis are:**

a. Pneumonia and severe pulmonary emphysema

b. Depression of respiratory centre

c. Left-sided heart failure

d. All of these

49. **Consider the following statements regarding acidemia. Which are true?**

i. Respiratory rate may be slower, depth of respiration is shallower than normal

ii. Tachycardia

iii. Amplitude of pulse and blood pressure both decrease

iv. Weakness, lassitude and terminal coma

a. i is true

b. i and ii are true

c. i, ii, and iii are true

d. All are true

50. **Which of the following are correct as causes of oedema?**

i. Decreased plasma oncotic pressure

ii. Increased hydrostatic pressure in capillaries and veins

iii. Increased capillary permeability

iv. Obstruction to lymphatic flow

a. i, ii, iii and iv

b. i and iii

c. i and ii

d. i, ii and iii

51. **The strong ion difference (SID) of ruminant plasma is approximately:**

    a. 10 meq/L

    b. 30 meq/L

    c. 20 meq/L

    d. 40 meq/L

52. **How much saliva can cattle produce per day?**

    a. 18 litres

    b. 100 litres

    c. 180 litres

    d. 80 litres

53. **The optimal oral electrolyte solution should have a sodium concentration between:**

    a. 90–130 mmol/L

    b. 9–13 mmol/L

    c. 70–90 mmol/L

    d. 10–30 mmol/L

54. **The normal plasma osmolality in ruminants is approximately:**

    a. 185 mOsm/kg

    b. 285 mOsm/kg

    c. 285 meq/L

    d. 85 mOsm/kg

55. **The insensible water loss in the neonatal calf is:**

    a. 5 ml/kg/d

    b. 35 ml/kg/d

    c. 15 ml/kg/d

    d. 25 ml/kg/d

56. **The optimal parenteral fluid for dehydrated ruminants is:**

a. Large volume hyperosmotic crystalloid solutions

b. Large volume hypo-osmotic crystalloid solutions

c. Large volume iso-osmotic crystalloid solutions

d. Crystalloid solutions

57. **Dehydrated or endotoxaemic neonatal ruminants typically have:**

a. Hyponatraemic, hyperkalaemic, metabolic acidosis

b. Hypenatraemic, hyperkalaemic, metabolic acidosis

c. Hypochloremic, hypokalaemic, metabolic alkalosis

d. None of the above

58. **Administration of large quantities of calcium gluconate or calcium borogluconate to ruminants induces a mild strong-ion acidosis. How would you respond to this statement?**

a. Ruminants do not metabolize gluconate

b. Ruminants metabolize gluconate and produce acidosis

c. Ruminants develop alkalosis

d. Ruminants metabolize gluconate and produce alkalosis

59. **The preferred sample for hypomagnesemic tetany in cattle is:**

a. Serum

b. CSF

c. Plasma

d. Urine

60. **The normal cardiac response to calcium administration in cattle is:**

a. Increase in the strength of cardiac contraction

b. Slowing of the heart rate

c. a and b

d. None of these

61. **Which magnesium concentration (mmol/l) of CSF will show the signs of tetany in hypomagnesemia?**

    a. 0.4

    b. 0.04

    c. 4

    d. 1

62. **Dehydrated or endotoxaemic adult ruminants typically have:**

    a. Hyponatraemic, hyperkalaemic, metabolic acidosis

    b. Hypochloremic, hyperkalaemic, metabolic alkalosis

    c. Hyponatraemic, hypokalaemic, metabolic acidosis

    d. Hypochloremic, hypokalaemic, metabolic alkalosis

63. **A useful form of phosphorus for treating hypophosphataemia in cattle is:**

    a. Phosphites

    b. Hypophosphite

    c. Calcium hypophosphite

    d. Phosphates

64. **How many ml of 23% calcium borogluconate/kg body weight/ min is the maximum safe rate of calcium administration in cattle?**

    a. 0.065 ml

    b. 1 ml

    c. 0.65 ml

    d. 0.0065 ml

65. **Salivary phosphorus production in ruminants is between:**

    a. 25 to 100 g/day

    b. 25 to 50 g/day

    c. 50 to 100 g/day

    d. 25 to 75 g/day

66. **Calcium outflow increases by how many grams per day into the foetal skeleton prior to calving?**

    a. 10

    b. 20

    c. 30

    d. 5

67. **Which two symptoms play a role in paradoxic aciduria?**

    a. Hypovolaemia, hyponatraemia

    b. Hypovolaemia, hypokalaemia

    c. Hypovolaemia, hypochloraemia

    d. Hypovolaemia, hypocalcaemia

68. **What is the formula for total base replacement need?**

    a. Acid deficit x 0.3 x Body weight

    b. Base deficit x 0.3 x Body weight

    c. Base deficit x 0.2 x Body weight

    d. Acid deficit x 3.0 x Body weight

69. **Excretion of calcium in total colostrum is:**

    a. 10 g

    b. 30 g

    c. 20 g

    d. 5 g

70. **The blood concentration of parathyroid hormone in cows suffering from clinical milk fever is:**

    a. 500 pg/ml

    b. 2000 pg/ml

    c. 1500 pg/ml

    d. 1000 pg/ml

71. **Subcutaneous administration of calcium solutions to facilitate absorption should be:**

   a. Not more than 15 ml at a site

   b. Not more than 25 ml at a site

   c. Not more than 125 ml at a site

   d. Not more than 105 ml at a site

72. **The most aggressive intravenous treatment protocol for hypokalaemia is 1.15% KCl, which should be administered at:**

   a. Less than 3.2 ml/kg/h

   b. Less than 1.2 ml/kg/h

   c. Less than 3.2 ml/kg/min

   d. Less than 2.2 ml/kg/h

73. **Fatal arrhythmia begins at a blood calcium concentration of:**

   a. 3–4 mmol/L

   b. 4–5 mmol/L

   c. 7–8 mmol/L

   d. 5–6 mmol/L

74. **Rebound hypocalcaemia following IV calcium administration is caused by the combined effects of:**

   a. PTH and CT

   b. Impaired PTH secretion and increased calcitonin

   c. Increased PTH and decreased CT

   d. None of these

75. **Which route of fluid therapy has been classically used to correct hydro-electrolytic and acid-base imbalances in adult ruminants due to its effectiveness and practicality?**

   a. Intravenous

   b. Subcutaneous

   c. Intra-osseous

   d. Enteral

76. Which organ acts in the elimination of excess acids and bases of non-respiratory origin, playing a fundamental role in the maintenance of the acid–base balance?

   a. Liver

   b. Stomach

   c. Kidneys

   d. Lungs

77. The primary route of fluid administration in small ruminants is/are:

   a. Oral route

   b. Intravenous route

   c. Neither a nor b

   d. Both a and b

78. The most common cause of ongoing fluid loss in small ruminants is:

   a. Acidosis

   b. Diarrhoea

   c. Saliva loss

   d. Polyuria

79. In severely dehydrated and/or hypovolemic animals, a 'shock dose' for sheep and goats is:

   a. 10–20 ml/kg

   b. 30–40 ml/kg

   c. 50–80 ml/kg

   d. 20–50 ml/kg

80. Crystalloid fluids can be classified as:

   a. Isotonic, hypotonic or hypertonic

   b. Isotonic

   c. Hypertonic

   d. Hypotonic

81. **Which crystalloids contain an osmolarity (mOsm/L) that is similar to extracellular fluid?**

    a. Hypotonic

    b. Isotonic

    c. Hypertonic

    d. None of these

82. **Plasma is recommended at what dose for neonates with failure of passive transfer (FPT)?**

    a. 10–20 ml/kg

    b. 10–30 ml/kg

    c. 5–10 ml/kg

    d. 20 –40 ml/kg

83. **Whole blood transfusions are recommended in small ruminants when the PCV is at what level in cases of chronic anaemia, and at what level in cases of acute anaemia?**

    a. $\leq 12\%, \leq 15\%$

    b. $\leq 12\%, \leq 10\%$

    c. $\leq 15\%, \leq 12\%$

    d. $\leq 10\%, \leq 15\%$

84. **Which type of hypersensitivity reaction develops during whole-blood transfusion?**

    a. Type II

    b. Type III

    c. Type I

    d. None of these

85. **In small ruminants, as a general rule of thumb, the donor can safely donate how much blood at one time?**

    a. 10 ml/kg

    b. 15 ml/kg

    c. 20 ml/kg

    d. 1 ml/kg

86. **Oral electrolyte solutions can be made by adding the following, per litre of water:**

    a. 7 g NaCl, 1.5 g KCl and 0.5 g $CaCl_2$

    b. 1.5 g NaCl, 7 g KCl and 0.5 g $CaCl_2$

    c. Neither a nor b

    d. 0.5 g NaCl, 1.5 g KCl and 7 g $CaCl_2$

87. **Which test is used to identify hydration status by tenting?**

    a. Capillary refill time

    b. Skin lifting test

    c. Skin turgor test

    d. None of these

88. **Tall T waves in an ECG are indicative of:**

    a. Hyperkalaemia

    b. Hypokalaemia

    c. Hypocalcaemia

    d. Hypoglycaemia

89. **A prolonged ST interval in an ECG is indicative of:**

    a. Hyperkalaemia

    b. Hypokalaemia

    c. Hypocalcaemia

    d. Hypoglycaemia

90. **Hypokalaemia in cattle occurs in the following conditions except:**

    a. Caecal dilatation

    b. Abomasal impaction

    c. Right-side displacement of abomasums

    d. Abomasal torsion

91. **Hypokalaemia occurs in cattle following repeated administration of:**

    a. Isoflupredone acetate

    b. Fludocortisone

    c. Dexamethasone

    d. Betamethasone

92. **The normal serum potassium level in cattle is:**

    a. 2–3 meq/L

    b. 3.2–4.3 meq/L

    c. 3.9–5.8 meq/L

    d. 5.5.–26 meq/L

93. **What is the dose and percentage of intravenous potassium chloride?**

    a. 0.5 mmol/kg and 1.15%

    b. 0.75 mmol/kg and 1.5%

    c. 1.0 mmol/kg and 2.2%

    d. 1.1 mmol/kg and 2.3%

94. **The classical symptoms of hypokalemia are:**

    a. Muscle weakness

    b. Recumbency

    c. Anorexia

    d. All of these

95. **The oral dose of potassium chloride for treatment of hypokalaemia in cattle is:**

    a. 30–60 g

    b. 60–120 g

    c. 120–240 g

    d. 250–300 g

96. **High dose of intravenous potassium chloride is lethal in cattle in case of:**

    a. Cardiac arrhythmia

    b. Ventricular fibrillation

    c. a and b

    d. None of these

97. **Increased dose of oral potassium chloride is not recommended for ruminants because it causes:**

    a. Diarrhoea

    b. Salivation and muscle tremor

    c. Excitability

    d. All of these

98. **The major organ involved in magnesium homeostasis is :**

    a. Liver

    b. Bones

    c. Kidney

    d. Intestine

99. **The normal serum magnesium level in cattle is:**

    a. 1.2–1.6 mg/dl

    b. 1.8–2.3 mg/dl

    c. 2.2–3.1 mg/dl

    d. 3.1–4.4 mg/dl

100. **Hypomagnesaemia is also called:**

    a. Lactation tetany

    b. Grass staggers

    c. Wheat pasture poisoning

    d. All of these

101. **What is the concentration of magnesium in CSF of cattle with lactation tetany?**

    a. 1.25 mg/dl

    b. 1.32 mg/dl

    c. 1.42 mg/dl

    d. 1.50 mg/dl

102. **What are the classical symptoms of hypomagnesemia in calves?**

    a. Shaking of the head

    b. Hyperesthesia

    c. Convulsions

    d. All of these

103. **Hypomagnesemic tetany in calves is often complicated by:**

    a. Ketosis

    b. Copper deficiency

    c. Enzootic muscular dystrophy

    d. a and c

104. **Statement I: The serum magnesium concentration in cattle is influenced by the Na:K ratio in the rumen.**
    Statement II: Absorption of magnesium is determined by dietary and salivary concentration of sodium and potassium.
    Consider the following statements:

    a. Both I and II are correct

    b. Both I and II are incorrect

    c. I correct, II incorrect

    d. I incorrect, II correct

105. **Statement I: Increased concentration of potassium and nitrogen in the diet reduces absorption of magnesium and calcium**
Statement II: Rapidly growing young grasses have high potassium and depress the Na:K ratio. Consider the following statements:

   a. Both I and II are correct

   b. Both I and II are incorrect

   c. I correct, II incorrect

   d. I incorrect, II correct

106. **Hypomagnesemia is common in which season?**

   a. Summer

   b. Spring

   c. Winter

   d. Autumn

107. **High content of what in pasture affects magnesium absorption?**

   a. Potassium

   b. Nitrogen

   c. Sodium

   d. Manganese

108. **Low intake of magnesium and hyperactivity of the thyroid gland occurs in which season?**

   a. Summer

   b. Spring

   c. Winter

   d. Autumn

109. **A sudden rise of concentration of what in the rumen impairs magnesium absorption?**

    a. Phosphorus

    b. Ammonia

    c. Potassium

    d. Nitrogen

110. **Which of these reduces the production and secretion of PTH and hydroxylation of vitamin D in the liver?**

    a. Phosphorus deficiency

    b. Calcium deficiency

    c. Hypomagnesemia

    d. Manganese deficiency

111. **Chronic subclinical hypomagnesemia increases susceptibility to:**

    a. Tetanic convulsions

    b. Milk fever

    c. Neither a nor b

    d. PPH

112. **Primary phosphorus deficiency in the diet is characterized by:**

    a. Pica

    b. Poor growth rate

    c. Infertility

    d. All of these

113. **Which is a common finding of hypophosphataemia in horses?**

    a. Chronic renal failure

    b. Liver failure

    c. Osteodystrophy

    d. None of these

114. **Primary phosphorus deficiency is common in:**

    a. Cattle

    b. Horses

    c. Pigs

    d. Goats

115. **The intravenous infusion of large quantities of fluids and electrolytes is a high priority in the management of**

    a. Endotoxemia

    b. Parasitic infection

    c. Burn injury

    d. None of these

116. **For treatment of endotoxic shock, large volumes of which fluid have been preferred?**

    a. Isotonic

    b. Any crystalloids

    c. Colloids

    d. Plasma

117. **The vasopressor agent of choice in hypotensive animals is**

    a. Lidocaine

    b. Norepinephrine

    c. Dobutamine

    d. Dopamine

118. **Excess loss of phosphorus in phospholipids of milk following onset of lactation leads to:**

    a. PPH

    b. Hypocalcaemia

    c. Low fat syndrome

    d. All of these

119. **The major gluconeogenic precursor in sheep is:**

   a. Propionate

   b. Butyrate

   c. Amino acid

   d. a and c

120. **The precipitating factor for pregnancy toxaemia in sheep is:**

   a. Plasma cortisol

   b. Hepatic dysfunction

   c. BHBA

   d. a and b

121. **The most common clinical manifestation of pregnancy toxaemia in sheep is:**

   a. Hypoglycaemic encephalopathy

   b. Hyperglycaemic encephalopathy

   c. Hepatic encephalopathy

   d. None of these

122. **The most commonly used gluconeogenic precursor for treatment of pregnancy toxaemia in sheep is:**

   a. Glycerine

   b. Propylene glycol

   c. Citrate

   d. a and b

123. **Which major biochemical changes occur in pregnancy toxaemia?**

   a. Ketonemia

   b. Metabolic acidosis

   c. Uraemia

   d. All of these

124. **A good indicator of negative energy balance in sheep is:**

a. BHBA

b. Ketone

c. Acetone

d. NEFA

125. **Which of the following are classical symptoms of pregnancy toxaemia in sheep?**

a. Blindness

b. Circling

c. Dorsiflexion of the head

d. All of these

126. **Pregnancy toxaemia in ewes mostly occurs in the last _____ weeks of gestation:**

a. 1–2

b. 2–3

c. 2–4

d. 0–1

127. **In pregnant ewes, the percentage of foetal growth that occurs in the last 6 weeks of gestation is:**

a. 90%

b. 80%

c. 60%

d. 70%

128. **Which of the following reduces the degree of ionization of serum calcium?**

a. Neomycin

b. Zinc oxide

c. Endotoxin

d. All of these

129. Which of the following in a prepartum diet decreases the incidence of milk fever?

a. Calcium and phosphorus

b. Sodium and potassium

c. Sulphate and chloride

d. Magnesium and potassium

130. Which of the following organs are involved in the regulation of the calcium homeostatic mechanism?

a. Parathyroid gland

b. Bone

c. Kidneys

d. All of these

131. Parturient paresis in sheep mostly occurs in:

a. Prepartum period

b. Periparturient period

c. Pre- and postparturient periods

d. Postparturient period

132. Hypocalcaemia in cattle predisposes to:

a. Left-side displacement of abomasum

b. Right-side displacement of abomasum

c. Abomasal torsion

d. Caecal dilatation

133. Hypocalcaemia in late pregnant ewes could induce:

a. Neonatal hyperthyroidism

b. Neonatal hypoglycaemia

c. Hypoinsulinemia

d. a and c

134. **'Feeding excess calcium and phosphorus during prepartum decreases the incidence of milk fever.' Is this statement:**

a. Correct

b. Incorrect

c. More common in pre-partum

d. Most common in postpartum

135. **Impact of feeding low calcium- and phosphorus-containing diet to ruminants during the prepartum period:**

a. Increases intestinal absorption and mobilization from bones

b. Decreases intestinal absorption and mobilization from bones

c. Increases intestinal absorption of calcium only

d. Increases mobilization of calcium from bones

136. **Which condition causes atony of the plain and cardiac muscles?**

a. Hypercalcaemia

b. Hypomagnesaemia

c. Hypocalcaemia

d. Hypokalaemia

137. **The condition that interferes with the release of acetylcho-line at the neuromuscular junction is:**

a. Hypokalaemia

b. Hypocalcaemia

c. Hyponatraemia

d. Hypercalcaemia

138. **The occurrence of hypocalcaemia in sheep is mostly:**

a. Sporadic

b. Single case

c. a and b

d. Outbreak

139. **Hypocalcaemia occurs in cows in the stage of:**

   a. Oestrus

   b. Anoestrus

   c. Pro-oestrus

   d. All of these

140. **An elevated level of which of the following hormone in the blood depresses the appetite centre?**

   a. Progesterone

   b. Cortisol

   c. Oestrogen

   d. b and c

141. **Addition of ammonium chloride in the diet of pregnant animals during the prepartum period:**

   a. Reduces the chances of milk fever

   b. Has no effect on milk fever

   c. Increases the chance of milk fever

   d. Increases feed intake

142. **The serum level of which component is a good indicator of hepatic functionality in cattle?**

   a. Potassium

   b. Glucose

   c. Calcium

   d. Liver enzymes

143. **Which of the following aids in the estimation of total lipids and triglycerides in cows with fatty liver?**

   a. Serum

   b. Tissue biopsy

   c. Liver biopsy

   d. Plasma estimates

144. **What is the effect that DCAD method has on cows during late prepartum and early postpartum periods?**

    a. Decreases the blood pH

    b. Increases the blood pH

    c. Balances the blood pH

    d. None of these

145. **Which readily absorbable substance is added to the diet to decrease the pH of the blood?**

    a. Anions salts

    b. Cationic salts

    c. a and b

    d. None of these

146. **DCAD reduces blood pH by reducing which ion in the diet?**

    a. Calcium

    b. Sulfur

    c. Chloride

    d. Potassium

147. **The DCAD value for prevention of milk fever is:**

    a. −15 to +15 meq/100g of dry matter

    b. −25 to +25 meq/100g of dry matter

    c. −35 to +35 meq/100g of dry matter

    d. −45 to +45 meq/100g of dry matter

148. **In postparturient haemoglobinuria, crystalloid fluids may be administered to:**

    a. Protect the heart against toxic and anoxic damage

    b. Protect the kidneys against toxic and anoxic damage

    c. Protect the lungs against toxic and anoxic damage

    d. Protect the spleen against toxic and anoxic damage

149. **A fat to protein ratio greater than 1:5 in milk is indicative of:**

a. Ketosis

b. Hypocalcaemia

c. Protein losing enteropathy

d. Mastitis

150. **Which of the following is used to avoid relapses of primary ketosis in terms of treatment response?**

a. Corticosteroids and IV glucose

b. Corticosteroids

c. IV glucose

d. None of these

151. **Hypocalcaemia in milking goats is most common in the age group of:**

a. 4–6-years

b. 2–4 years

c. 2–6 years

d. 1–2 year

152. **In which condition do we see an increase in the cell membrane permeability of muscle fibres and loss of potassium from the cells in the downer cows, causing myotonia?**

a. Hypokalaemia

b. Hypocalcaemia

c. Hyperkalaemia

d. Hypoglycaemia

153. **Mineralocorticoids increase loss of potassium in the:**

a. Faeces

b. Saliva

c. Urine

d. None of these

154. **Mineralocorticoid activity enhances which type of tubular secretion of potassium?**

   a. Proximal

   b. Distal

   c. Collecting

   d. a and b

155. **Which of these is the state-of-the-art treatment for critically ill ruminants?**

   a. Parenteral nutrition

   b. Enteral nutrition

   c. Non-parenteral nutrition

   d. None of these

156. **What is shock?**

   a. Acute circulatory failure

   b. Volume overload

   c. Pressure overload

   d. b and c

157. **What can result from changes in pH, K^+, and Na^+ or decreased Ca^{2+}?**

   a. Depression and inappetence

   b. Mania

   c. Excitement

   d. Muscular weakness

158. **Which substance forms a true solution and is capable of being crystallized?**

   a. Colloids

   b. Plasma volume expanders

   c. Crystalloids

   d. a and b

159. **What may be associated with changes in pH, K⁺ and Na?**

   a. Depression and inappetence

   b. Mania

   c. Excitement

   d. Muscular weakness

160. **Which substance is a 'classic crystalloid' because table salt exists as a crystal but dissolves completely when placed in water?**

   a. NaCl

   b. KCl

   c. Sodium bicarbonate

   d. a and b

161. **Sodium-containing crystalloid solutions also are contraindicated in the presence of severe**

   a. Hypoalbuminemia

   b. Hyperalbuminemia

   c. a and b

   d. None of these

162. **Sodium-containing crystalloid solutions are always indicated in what?**

   a. Hypovolaemia

   b. Hypervolaemia

   c. Hypoalbuminaemia

   d. Shock

163. **In veterinary and human medicine, crystalloid solutions are expressed more frequently in terms of the number of what, per volume of solution?**

   a. Ionised portions

   b. Non-Ionised portions

c. Charged components

d. Non-charged components

164. **Electrolyte solutions with an effective SID level of what are acidifying, because they create a strong-ion acidosis?**

a. Less than 0

b. Equal to 0

c. Greater than 0

d. None of these

165. **What term is used to describe the number of dissolved particles per kg of solution, expressed as mOsm/kg?**

a. SID

b. Osmolarity

c. Osmolality

d. Tonicity

166. **What term is used to describe the number of particles per litre of solution, expressed as mOsm/l?**

a. Osmolarity

b. Osmolality

c. SID

d. Tonicity

167. **Normal plasma osmolality of 285 mOsm/kg is equivalent to a plasma water osmolarity of _____**

a. 306 mOsm/kg

b. 285 mOsm/g

c. 306 mOsm/L

d. 285 mOsm/L

168. **Plasma ISO osmolarity for ruminants is:**

a. > 312 mOsm/L

b. < 312 mOsm/L

  c. 300–312 mOsm/L

  d. < 300 mOsm/L

169. **How do ruminant erythrocytes react to increases in plasma osmolarity?**

  a. They are fragile to it

  b. They are resistant to it

  c. They are susceptible to it

  d. None of these

170. **The plasma hypo-osmolarity for ruminants is:**

  a. > 312 mOsm/L

  b. < 312 mOsm/L

  c. 300–312 mOsm/L

  d. < 300 mOsm/L

171. **Water moves across the semipermeable red blood cell membrane into the erythrocyte, resulting in swelling of erythrocytes, rupture of the cell membrane and haemolysis as the osmolarity of the solution:**

  a. Increases

  b. Is equalized

  c. Decreases

  d. a and b

172. **Rapid ingestion of large volumes of water in neonatal and adult ruminants causes:**

  a. Haemolysis

  b. Haemoglobinuria

  c. a and b

  d. None of these

173. **Increasing plasma osmolarity causes water to move out of erythrocytes, which are resistant to:**

    a. Haemoglobinuria

    b. Shrinking

    c. Haemolysis

    d. None of these

174. **A solution that is similar to the osmolality of plasma that will cause no cell damage, is called:**

    a. Normal Saline

    b. Hypotonic

    c. Isotonic

    d. Hypertonic

175. **Which of the following is a balanced, polyionic, alkalinizing, isosmotic, crystalloid solution containing physiologic concentrations of Na^+, K^+, Ca^{2+}, Cl^- and lactate?**

    a. Ringer's lactate

    b. Normal saline

    c. a and b

    d. Lactated Ringer's solution

176. **Lactated Ringer's solution alkalinizes because lactate is metabolized predominantly to:**

    a. Hydrogen Ion

    b. L-lactate

    c. Bicarbonate ion

    d. None of these

177. **Lactate in lactated Ringer's solution is a racemic what of L-lactate and D-lactate?**

    a. Equimolar mixture

    b. Hypomolar mixture

c. Hypermolar mixture

d. b and c

178. **Which of these can also be used in gluconeogenesis instead of bicarbonate production?**

a. D-lactate

b. L-lactate

c. DL-lactate

d. None of these

179. **Which dehydrogenase activity is negligible in ruminant tissues?**

a. D-lactate

b. L-lactate

c. DL-lactate

d. None of these

180. **The rate of lactate metabolism to glucose is decreased by approximately how much in severely dehydrated calves?**

a. 100%

b. 50%

c. 25%

d. 90%

181. **Acetated Ringer's solution contains which substance(s) which, like D-lactate, is metabolized poorly by neonatal calves?**

a. Gluconate

b. Gluconate and lactate

c. Lactate

d. None of these

182. **Which of these provides an alternative alkalinizing agent to NaHCO$_3$?**

a. Tris-hydroxymethyl aminomethane

b. Tham

c. Tromethamine

d. All of these

183. **After administration, what percentage of neutral compound in tromethamine is protonated immediately to the strong cation in plasma?**

a. 90%

b. 70%

c. 50%

d. 80%

184. **What percentage of the administered tromethamine remains unprotonated and therefore can cross cell membranes and potentially buffer the intracellular compartment?**

a. 70%

b. 50%

c. 30%

d. 40%

185. **Which of these is an experimental iso-osmotic buffer (300 mOsm/L), made from equimolar disodium carbonate and NaHCO$_3$?**

a. Carbicarb

b. Acidecarb

c. Tham

d. Tham-E

186. **Like Ringer's solution, which of these is mildly acidifying because effective SID equals 0 mRq/L?**

a. 0.9% NaCl

b. 0.45% NaCl

c. None of these

d. a and b

187. **Which is hyponatraemic, hyperkaliaemic and hyperlactataemic, and does not contain calcium or magnesium?**

    a. Tris-hydroxymethyl aminomethane

    b. Darrow's solution

    c. Tromethamine

    d. a and b

188. **Which iso-osmotic polyionic solution was formulated for intravenous and intraperitoneal administration to dehydrated diarrhoeic calves?**

    a. McSherry's balanced electrolyte solution

    b. Darrow's solution

    c. a and b

    d. None of these

189. **Which solution is approximately 8 times normal osmolarity?**

    a. 20% dextrose

    b. 25% dextrose

    c. 50% dextrose

    d. 10% dextrose

190. **Hypertonic saline should be administered at what concentration intravenously per kg bodyweight for 4 to 5 minutes?**

    a. 4–5 ml/kg

    b. 1–2ml/kg

    c. 3–4 ml/kg

    d. None of these

191. **Hypertonic saline should be administered at what concentration?**

    a. 4 ml/kg/min

    b. 5 ml/kg/min

    c. 1 ml/kg/min

    d. 2 ml/kg/min

192. **Faster rates of 7.2% sodium chloride administration lead to what, due to vasodilation and decreased cardiac contractility?**

   a. Mild SID

   b. Haemodynamic collapse

   c. a and b

   d. None of these

193. **The speed of intravenous administration of 8.4% NaHCO$_3$ should not exceed:**

   a. 4 ml/kg/min

   b. 5 ml/kg/min

   c. 2 ml/kg/min

   d. 1 ml/kg/min

194. **The speed of intravenous administration of 5.0% NaHCO$_3$ should not exceed:**

   a. 4 ml/kg/min

   b. 5 ml/kg/min

   c. 2 ml/kg/min

   d. 1 ml/kg/min

195. **Calcium gluconate should not be added to NaHCO$_3$ solutions because which precipitate forms immediately, which interferes with normal fluid administration?**

   a. Yellow precipitate

   b. White precipitate

   c. a and b

   d. None of these

196. **Calcium gluconate should not be administered with tetracycline antibiotics because of the formation of which precipitate?**

   a. Yellow

   b. White

c. a and b

d. None of these

197.   **Which solution is excellent for sustained expansion of plasma volume, in marked contrast to the effect of crystalloid solutions?**

a. Hypotonic

b. Isotonic

c. Colloid

d. Crystalloid

198.   **Colloid solutions are contraindicated in which condition because these animals have increased plasma volume?**

a. Congestive heart failure

b. Cirrhosis

c. Acidosis

d. All of these

199.   **Colloid solutions are contraindicated in the presence of oliguric or anuric renal failure because the sustained volume overload may lead to what?**

a. CHF

b. Glomerulonephritis

c. Pulmonary oedema

d. None of these

200.   **Which of these is a perfectly balanced colloid–crystalloid solution, with great oxygen-carrying capacity?**

a. Stroma-free haemoglobin

b. Purified haemoglobin glutamer-200

c. Whole blood

d. None of these

Answers

1.	b	31.	b	61.	a	91.	a
2.	d	32.	d	62.	d	92.	c
3.	c	33.	a	63.	d	93.	a
4.	d	34.	b	64.	a	94.	d
5.	b	35.	a	65.	a	95.	b
6.	b	36.	d	66.	a	96.	c
7.	b	37.	b	67.	a	97.	d
8.	a	38.	d	68.	b	98.	c
9.	b	39.	c	69.	b	99.	b
10.	a	40.	d	70.	b	100.	d
11.	b	41.	b	71.	c	101.	a
12.	a	42.	a	72.	a	102.	d
13.	b	43.	a	73.	c	103.	c
14.	c	44.	b	74.	b	104.	a
15.	a	45.	d	75.	d	105.	a
16.	b	46.	a	76.	c	106.	c
17.	d	47.	a	77.	d	107.	b
18.	c	48.	d	78.	b	108.	c
19.	b	49.	d	79.	c	109.	b
20.	a	50.	a	80.	a	110.	c
21.	b	51.	d	81.	b	111.	b
22.	c	52.	c	82.	d	112.	d
23.	d	53.	a	83.	a	113.	a
24.	b	54.	b	84.	c	114.	a
25.	a	55.	d	85.	b	115.	a
26.	d	56.	c	86.	a	116.	a
27.	b	57.	a	87.	c	117.	b
28.	a	58.	a	88.	a	118.	a
29.	b	59.	b	89.	c	119.	d
30.	a	60.	c	90.	a	120.	d

(Continued)

121.	a	141.	a	161.	a	181.	a
122.	d	142.	b	162.	a	182.	d
123.	d	143.	c	163.	c	183.	b
124.	a	144.	a	164.	b	184.	c
125.	d	145.	a	165.	c	185.	a
126.	c	146.	d	166.	a	186.	a
127.	b	147.	a	167.	c	187.	b
128.	d	148.	b	168.	c	188.	a
129.	c	149.	a	169.	b	189.	c
130.	d	150.	a	170.	d	190.	a
131.	c	151.	a	171.	c	191.	c
132.	a	152.	a	172.	c	192.	b
133.	d	153.	c	173.	b	193.	d
134.	b	154.	b	174.	c	194.	c
135.	a	155.	b	175.	d	195.	b
136.	c	156.	a	176.	c	196.	a
137.	b	157.	d	177.	a	197.	c
138.	d	158.	c	178.	b	198.	a
139.	a	159.	a	179.	a	199.	c
140.	c	160.	a	180.	b	200.	c

4 Diseases of the Respiratory System

Vipin Maurya and Jigyasa Rana

Introduction

The respiratory system includes the upper airway (nostrils, nasal cavity, sinuses, nasopharynx, larynx and trachea) and lower airway (bronchi, bronchioles and alveoli). The nose facilitates olfaction and temperature regulation in homeothermic individuals. The primary function of the respiratory system is to deliver oxygen to the lungs to be exchanged with carbon dioxide. In the majority of species, gaseous exchange occurs in the alveoli. Any dysfunction in the gaseous exchange in response to disease leads to respiratory distress. In addition, the system maintains acid-base balance, acts as a blood reservoir, destroys emboli, metabolizes certain bioactive substances (e.g. serotonin, prostaglandins, corticosteroids and leukotrienes), and activates angiotensin. Tortuosity of the nasal passages, presence of hair, cilia, and mucus, the cough reflex and bronchoconstriction all provide defence against invasion by microorganisms and other foreign particles by acting as primary barriers.

Physiological variations exist between different species. Cattle are prone to retrograde drainage from the pharynx, pulmonary hypertension and reduced ventilation during the winter. In addition, cattle have relatively smaller lungs with low tidal volume and functional residual capacity, and are more sensitive to changes in environmental temperatures than other species. These anatomic and physiologic differences largely determine why some pathogens affect only some species (e.g. *Mannheimia haemolytica* affects cattle but not pigs) and why pneumonia is very important in some species (cattle, pigs) but less so in others (dogs, cats).

An animal with hypoxia shows signs of respiratory distress. Reduced oxygen-carrying capacity of the blood due to anaemic hypoxia (caused by a decreased number of red blood cells), hypoperfusion (by decreased cardiac output), anatomic shunt, physiologic shunt, decreased inhaled oxygen,

© CAB International 2024. *Key Questions in Clinical Farm Animal Medicine Volume 1: Principles of Disease Examination, Diagnosis and Management* (ed. T. Rana)
DOI: 10.1079/9781800624788.0004

ventilation/perfusion mismatch, diffusion impairment, hypoventilation (e.g. hypoxic hypoxia), inability of tissues to use available oxygen (e.g. histotoxic hypoxia, as in cyanide poisoning) may all be the cause of hypoxia.

Congenital anomalies of the respiratory tract such as cysts in the sinuses and turbinates, tracheal hypoplasia, nasopharyngeal turbinates and accessory lungs are rare but do occur. A common cause of upper respiratory tract malfunction is rhinitis (which results in serous exudate with the presence of few neutrophils and macrophages, erosion and ulceration of the nasal mucosa). It may be caused by viruses, bacteria, fungi, parasites and hypersensitivity reactions, such as localized allergies and anaphylaxis.

Laryngitis, tracheitis and bronchitis result in coughing and possibly inspiratory or expiratory dyspnoea. One of the most common respiratory diseases is pneumonia, which is defined as inflammation of the lungs. There are many ways to classify the various types of pneumonia. The most commonly used classification is on the basis of distribution of lesions. Focal pneumonia has one or more discrete foci in a random pattern (e.g. abscessation due to emboli from other sites, tuberculosis or actinomycosis). Lobular pneumonia accentuates the anatomic pattern of lobules (e.g. bronchopneumonia caused by *Pasteurella multocida*. Lobar pneumonia affects large areas of lobes and is often severe (e.g. fibrinous pneumonic pasteurellosis of cattle). Diffuse or interstitial pneumonia often involve the entire lung. Bacterial proliferation occurs due to breakdown of the host defence mechanism as a result of stress (e.g. transportation, concurrent illness) or cellular insult (e.g. viral infection, toxicity). These bacteria may overwhelm the normal defence mechanisms, localize, multiply and initiate inflammation. Some respiratory viral infections can cause temporary dysfunction of phagocytic mechanisms of the alveolar macrophages. This usually occurs several days after viral exposure. Inhaled bacteria proliferate and pneumonia ensues, often with an overwhelming infection and massive exudation into the alveoli.

Pneumonia can also be caused by viral, bacterial and fungal infection and toxins arriving hematogenously, by inhalation, or by aspiration of food or gastric contents. Bronchiectasis is a chronic lesion of the bronchi and parenchyma characterized by irreversible cylindrical or saccular dilatation, secondary infection and atelectasis. Ulceration of bronchioles caused by a virus may lead to formation of organized plugs of connective tissue in the small bronchioles, a lesion called bronchiolitis obliterans, which may cause permanent obstruction, atelectasis and severe respiratory insufficiency.

Most infectious pneumonias develop in the anteroventral portions of the lungs. However, infectious agents, as well as malignant tumour cells, can invade the lungs via the bloodstream. Fluid or air within the pleural space (i.e. empyema, hydrothorax, chylothorax, atelectasis, diaphragmatic hernia or pneumothorax) can also seriously impair respiratory function.

Pulmonary thrombosis is a serious condition which leads to acute, often fulminant, respiratory failure as a result of a lack of pulmonary arterial blood flow to ventilated regions of the lungs.

In cases of respiratory distress, the affected animals prefer to be in a standing position instead of lying down, or lie only in sternal recumbency, or may assume a sitting position (also known as orthopnoea). Auscultation of the chest may reveal crackles or rales in cases of pneumonia. Diseases associated with pleura mainly occur due to accumulation of fluid or air in the pleural sac, leading to respiratory distress. Short, choppy breathing with an increase in the rate and effort is usually seen, often with paradoxical movement of the chest and abdomen with each breath. Pleuritis (pleurisy) may be caused by any pathogen that gains entrance to the pleural cavity, and can be an extension of bronchopneumonia. Rapid, shallow breathing, fever and thoracic pain are suggestive of pleuritis. Auscultation of the chest may reveal friction sounds as well as dull lung sounds.

Multiple Choice Questions

1. **Glanders is caused by:**

   a. *Mycobacterium* spp.

   b. *Burkholderia/Pseudomonas* spp.

   c. *Staphylococcus* spp.

   d. *Streptococcus* spp.

2. **Laboratory cultivation of *Rhinosporidium seeberii* can be performed in:**

   a. Cornmeal agar

   b. Sabouraud's dextrose agar

   c. Potato agar

   d. None of these

3. **In horses, light-red foam coming from both nostrils and harsh sounds over the trachea and bronchi indicates:**

   a. Pulmonary haemorrhage

   b. Pharyngeal haemorrhage

   c. Nasal haemorrhage

   d. Pulmonary congestion

4. **To avoid collapse of the lungs upon closure of a thoracotomy, the surgeon's primary concern should be:**

   a. Suturing the intercostal muscles adequately

   b. Suturing the lateral thoracic musculature adequately

   c. Making sure the lung is moist before closure

   d. Creating negative pressure in the pleural cavity

5. **Following infection of cattle, *Dictyocaulus viviparous* larvae reach the lungs via the:**

   a. Intestine, portal vein, liver, heart, lungs

   b. Intestine, abdominal cavity, liver, heart, lungs

    c. Intestine, lymphatics, mesenteric lymph node, thoracic duct, heart, lungs

    d. Intestine, abdominal cavity, thoracic duct, heart, lungs

6. **Pneumonia caused by faulty drenching of medicine is called:**

    a. Aspiration pneumonia

    b. Suppurative pneumonia

    c. Intestinal pneumonia

    d. Granulomatous pneumonia

7. **'Brown induration' of the lungs is seen in:**

    a. Left-sided heart failure

    b. Right-sided heart failure

    c. a and b

    d. None of these

8. **In chronic venous congestion, the lungs are affected in:**

    a. Left-sided heart failure

    b. Right-sided heart failure

    c. a and b

    d. None of these

9. **Gangrene in the lungs is commonly caused by:**

    a. Asphyxia

    b. Epistaxis

    c. Faulty drenching

    d. Anaemia

10. **Deposition of silver dust in the lungs is called:**

    a. Acanthosis

    b. Chalicosis

    c. Anthracosis

    d. Argyrosis

11. **The commonest type of pneumonia in animals is:**

   a. Verminous pneumonia

   b. Bronchopneumonia

   c. Mycotic pneumonia

   d. All of these

12. **Suppuration is not encountered in tuberculosis because:**

   a. Calcification interferes with suppuration

   b. Caseous material in tuberculosis acts as an antienzyme

   c. Cord factor of mycobacteria interferes with suppuration

   d. All of these

13. **Dilatation and rupture of lung alveoli is called:**

   a. Atelectasis

   b. Bronchistenosis

   c. Bronchiectasis

   d. Emphysema

14. **Nasal polyps are caused by:**

   a. *Schistosoma nasalis*

   b. *Rhinosporidium seeberi*

   c. *E. coli*

   d. *Mycoplasma mycoides*

15. **Which type of pneumonia is seen in CCPP?**

   a. Verminous

   b. Broncho

   c. Mycotic

   d. Fibrinous

16. **Heaves or broken wind in horses is otherwise known as:**

   a. Acute alveolar emphysema

   b. Chronic interstitial pneumonia

c. Chronic alveolar emphysema

d. Acute bronchopneumonia

17. **The type of pneumonia seen in brooder pneumonia is:**

a. Fibrinous

b. Aspiration

c. Suppurative

d. Granulomatous

18. **'Marie's disease' is also known as:**

a. Pulmonary osteoarthropathy

b. Chondrodystrophia foetalis

c. Achondroplasia

d. None of these

19. **'Cells of tripier' are seen in the lungs during:**

a. Bronchopneumonia

b. Verminous pneumonia

c. Interstitial pneumonia

d. Mycotic pneumonia

20. **A common site for the metastasis for a primary tumour is:**

a. Lungs

b. Liver

c. Intestine

d. Brain

21. **Lung cancer can be contracted as a result of inhaling:**

a. Coal dust

b. Cement dust

c. Calcium fluoride

d. Bauxite dust

22. **The acute pulmonary form of African horse sickness is known as:**

   a. DUNKOP

   b. DIKKOP

   c. Mixed form

   d. None of these

23. **Infectious bovine rhinotracheitis is also known as:**

   a. Infectious pustular vulvovaginitis

   b. Coital exanthema

   c. Vesicular venereal disease

   d. All of these

24. **The presence of tubercles on pleura and mesentery is seen in:**

   a. Pearl disease

   b. Johne's disease

   c. Brucellosis

   d. Actinobacillosis

25. **Febrile viral disease with croupous pneumonia and diphtheritic inflammation of the GI tract is known as:**

   a. Swine fever

   b. Swine dysentery

   c. Swine septicaemia

   d. Fowl cholera

26. **Snuffles in rabbits is caused by:**

   a. *Clostridium piliformis*

   b. *Klebsiella pneumoniae*

   c. *Pasteurella multocida*

   d. *Bartonella bacilliformis*

27. **'Sequestra formation' and a marbled appearance of the lungs is characteristic of:**

   a. CBPP

   b. CCPP

   c. Tuberculosis

   d. a and b

28. **A marbled appearance of the lungs in adult cows is the characteristic post-mortem lesion of:**

   a. Contagious bovine pleuropneumonia

   b. Contagious caprine pleuropneumonia

   c. Strangles

   d. Tuberculosis

29. **Punched out ulcers in the mucosa of the trachea and larynx are seen in:**

   a. Glanders

   b. Farcy

   c. a and b

   d. None of these

30. **In poultry, an intradermal test for TB is performed in:**

   a. The skin

   b. The comb

   c. The wattle

   d. All of these

31. **Mycoplasmal disease of poultry is:**

   a. Chronic respiratory disease

   b. Chicken infectious anaemia

   c. Infectious coryza

   d. Avian encephalomyelitis

32. **Infectious laryngotracheitis is caused by:**

   a. Gallid Herpesvirus - 1

   b. Birnavirus

   c. Gallid Herpesvirus - 2

   d. Circovirus

33. **In the per acute form of infectious laryngotracheitis (ILT), the main lesion is:**

   a. Haemorrhagic tracheitis

   b. Caseous diphtheritic exudates

   c. Obstructive plugs in larynx

   d. All of these

34. **The presence of cheesy deposits in the air sacs is indicative of:**

   a. Infectious coryza

   b. Chronic respiratory disease

   c. Avian chlamydiosis

   d. Fowl spirochaetosis

35. **Caseous plug in the lower trachea and bronchi of dead chicks is observed in:**

   a. IBD

   b. EDS-76

   c. IB

   d. ILT

36. **The form of fowl pox causing high mortality in layers is:**

   a. Diphtheritic

   b. Dry

   c. Cutaneous

   d. None of these

37. **The main sign of ILT is:**

    a. Moist rales

    b. Breathing with a wide-open mouth and gasping

    c. Obstruction of the trachea with exudates

    d. All of these

38. **The first report of PPR was made in the Ivory Coast, West Africa, in which year**

    a. 1950

    b. 2001

    c. 1982

    d. 1942

39. **PPR virus has maximum affinity to:**

    a. Lymphoid tissues

    b. Respiratory cells

    c. Hepatic cells

    d. Renal cells

40. **Lungworm of cattle is:**

    a. *Dioctophyma renale*

    b. *Trichostrongylus axei*

    c. *Dictyocaulus viviparous*

    d. *Syngamus trachei*

41. **Which of the following worms causes verminous bronchitis in cattle?**

    a. *Parascaris equorum*

    b. *Dictyocaulus viviparous*

    c. *Dictyocaulus arnfieldi*

    d. *Dictyocaulus leucarti*

42. **Cloudiness, with the presence of cheesy exudates in the air sac membranes and body cavities, fibrinous pericarditis and perihepatitis, are lesions of:**

   a. Mycoplasmosis

   b. Avian Influenza

   c. Avian monocytosis

   d. Inclusion body hepatitis

43. **Multiple yellow-to-white pinpoint nodules scattered throughout the lung tissue is seen in:**

   a. Histoplasmosis

   b. Moniliasis

   c. Aspergillosis

   d. Favus

44. **Yellowish-white nodules (small bumps) in the lungs are characteristic of:**

   a. Aspergillosis

   b. Favus

   c. CRD

   d. Infectious coryza

45. **The bacterial strain used for the production of BCG vaccine is:**

   a. Nakayama

   b. PM-1503-3M

   c. 17-D

   d. Danish 1331

46. **Turkey coryza is caused by:**

   a. *Pasteurella aviseptica*

   b. *Bordetella avium*

   c. *Haemophilus paragallinarum*

   d. *Salmonella gallinarum*

47. **The mode of transmission for IBR virus is:**

   a. Venereal

   b. Inhalation

   c. Semen

   d. All of these

48. **Contagious caprine pleuropneumonia is caused by:**

   a. *Mycoplasma mycoides* subsp. *mycoides*

   b. *Mycoplasma mycoides* subsp. *capri*

   c. *Mycoplasma agalactiae*

   d. *Streptococcus pyogens*

49. **Suppurative bronchopneumonia and fibrinopurulent pleuritis in guinea pigs is caused by:**

   a. *Staphylococcus aureus*

   b. *Streptococcus pneumonia*

   c. *Streptococcus zooepidemicus*

   d. *Bordetella bronchiseptica*

50. **The organ of apparently healthy cattle that sheds *Pasteurella multocida* serotype B2 during periods of stress, is:**

   a. Tonsils

   b. Urinary bladder

   c. Vagina

   d. Mammary glands

51. **Diene's staining is used for:**

   a. *Mycoplasma*

   b. Bacteria

   c. Fungus

   d. Chlamydia

52. **Farmer's lung in cattle is caused by:**

a. *Micropolyspora faeni*

b. *Blastomyces bovis*

c. *Pithomyces chartarum*

d. *Histoplasma capsulatum*

53. **Chronic respiratory disease (CRD) in poultry is caused by:**

a. *Mycoplasma mycoides* subsp. *mycoides*

b. *Mycoplasma mycoides* subsp. *capri*

c. *Mycoplasma agalactiae*

d. *Mycoplasma gallisepticum*

54. **What is the name for the diagnostic test for tuberculosis in animals?**

a. Stormont test

b. Mantoux test

c. a and b

d. None of these

55. **Which medium is used for culture of *Mycoplasma*?**

a. PPLO agar

b. Frey's medium

c. a and b

d. Lowenstein Jensen medium

56. **Which condition is defined as 'insufficient oxygen to maintain normal metabolic functions'?**

a. Anoxia

b. Pneumonia

c. Anorexia

d. Hypoxia

57. **Hypoxia occurs when:**

    a. The brain is deficit in oxygen

    b. Arterial oxygen is 96 mmHg or less

    c. Arterial oxygen is 60 mmHg or less

    d. Arterial oxygen is less than 20 mmHg

58. **Coughing may be non-productive if the irritation is caused by:**

    a. Bacterial infections

    b. Viral infections

    c. Exudative infection

    d. Mucosal erosion

59. **Coughing is productive if caused by:**

    a. Copious exudate in the major airways

    b. Mucosal erosion

    c. Choking

    d. None of these

60. **Severe pulmonary oedema and emphysema can be caused by:**

    a. Respiratory insufficiency

    b. Anorexia

    c. Hyperthermia

    d. Rhinitis

61. **Which of the following is least likely to aid in the management and prevention of haemorrhagic septicaemia?**

    a. Increasing ventilation rate

    b. Reducing animal density

    c. Maintaining shed temperature between 32–35 °C.

    d. Decreasing humidity in the shed to 50%

62. **Mycobacterium tuberculosis, the usual cause of human tuberculosis:**

   a. Can infect bovines

   b. Infects only people

   c. Has a limited range of host

   d. Is typically destroyed by human saliva

63. **Advanced cases of bubaline tuberculosis not reacting to intradermal tuberculin testing are known as:**

   a. Anergic animals

   b. Photoallergic animals

   c. Visible lesions reactor (VLR)

   d. Exhausted animals

64. **Which of the following antibiotics is not effective against Mycoplasma?**

   a. Penicillin

   b. Tylosin

   c. Entamycin

   d. Oxytetracycline

65. **Nosocomial infections refer to:**

   a. Fatal infections

   b. Moderate infections

   c. Hospital-acquired infections

   d. Infections acquired through the nostrils

66. **Haemorrhagic septicaemia (HS) in buffalo is caused by:**

   a. Pasteurella multocida type E

   b. Pasteurella multocida type B

   c. Pasteurella multocida type C

   d. P. multocida type O

67. **The Glanders and Farcy Act was enacted in:**

   a. 1899

   b. 1999

   c. 1882

   d. 1985

68. **Canine parvovirus infection is best treated with:**

   a. Antibiotics + fluid therapy

   b. Steroids + fluid therapy

   c. Antibiotics + fluid therapy + granulocyte stimulating factor (filgrastim)

   d. Granulocyte stimulating factor alone

69. **CPR stands for:**

   a. Clinical practical performance

   b. Cardiac pulse recovery

   c. Cardiopulmonary resuscitation

   d. Cardiac pressure revival

70. **Inclusion bodies are found in RBCs in which condition?**

   a. Canine distemper

   b. Canine hepatitis

   c. Canine parvo

   d. Rabies

71. **Which respiratory sound can normally be detected without a stethoscope?**

   a. Vesicular

   b. Wheeze

   c. Stridor

   d. Crackle

72. **Pneumonia caused by aspiration of chemicals and drugs is called?**

    a. Fibrinous pneumonia

    b. Broncho pneumonia

    c. Drenching pneumonia

    d. Hypostatic Pneumonia

73. **Aspiration pneumonia is a common complication of what?**

    a. Stomatitis

    b. Pharyngitis

    c. Choke

    d. All of these

74. **Trypsin and chymotrypsin enzymes are useful in:**

    a. Acute pneumonia

    b. Bronchitis

    c. Drenching pneumonia

    d. Chronic pneumonia

75. **Vasoconstrictor drugs used in epistaxis include:**

    a. Adrenaline

    b. Alum

    c. Ice

    d. Vitamin C

76. **A common complication of pharyngitis is:**

    a. Bronchitis

    b. Laryngitis

    c. Aspiratory pneumonia

    d. Tracheitis

77. **_Rhodococcus equi_ is an important cause of a pyogranulomatous pneumonia in which group of horses?**

a. Stallions

b. Foals between 1 and 6 months of age

c. Colts

d. Mares

78. **The most serious cause of pneumonia in foals is:**

a. _Streptococcus equi_

b. _Rhodococcus equi_

c. _Streptococcus equi_

d. a and c

79. **Equine abortion virus infection is also called:**

a. Equine herpesvirus

b. Equine arteritis

c. Equine rhinopneumonitis

d. None of these

80. **Equine herpes virus infection is also called:**

a. Equine abortion virus

b. Equine arteritis

c. Equine rhinopneumonitis

d. None of these

81. **Both intracytoplasmic and intranuclear inclusions are present in:**

a. Rabies

b. Pox

c. Canine distemper

d. ICH

82. **In viral infections, the first cells to arrive are:**

a. Macrophages

b. Lymphocytes

c. Basophils

d. Neutrophils

83. **Pneumoconiosis is characterized by:**

a. Serous lesions in lungs

b. Fibrinous lesions in lungs

c. Haemorrhagic lesions in lungs

d. Granulomatous lesions in lungs

84. **Soft, productive, chronic cough usually originates from the:**

a. Pharynx

b. Larynx

c. Trachea

d. Lungs

85. **In highly pathogenic avian influenza virus, the multiple molecules of which amino acid are found at the cleavage site?**

a. Lysine

b. Arginine

c. Tryptophane

d. Serine

86. **A common term for deposition of exogenous substances in the body is:**

a. Anthracosis

b. Plumbism

c. Siderosis

d. Pneumoconiosis

87. **What are Opsonins?**

    a. Fc portion of IgG

    b. C3b fragment of complement

    c. Collectins

    d. All of the above

88. **A puppy presented with progressive weight loss, pneumonia and forced suckling with milk coming out from the nostrils is a good candidate for diagnosis of:**

    a. Salivary mucocele

    b. Cleft palate

    c. Megaoesophagus

    d. Choke

89. **The type of necrosis seen in hypoxic cell death is:**

    a. Caseative

    b. Liquifactive

    c. Fat necrosis

    d. Coagulative

90. **Accumulation of blood in the pleural sac is called:**

    a. Haemothorax

    b. Hydrothorax

    c. Pneumothorax

    d. Pyothorax

91. **Reduced supply of oxygen to the brain leads to:**

    a. Syncope

    b. Coma

    c. Epilepsy

    d. Cerebral oedema

92. **What term is used to describe decreased respiratory rate?**

   a. Apnoea

   b. Orthopnoea

   c. Oligopnoea

   d. Dyspnoea

93. **Accumulation of fluid in the thoracic cavity is known as:**

   a. Pneumothorax

   b. Hydrothorax

   c. a and b

   d. None of these

94. **Frequent dry cough, often in paroxysms, is seen in:**

   a. Bronchopneumonia

   b. Interstitial pneumonia

   c. Pneumonia

   d. Bronchitis

95. **Short, jerky inspiration caused by stimulation of the phrenic nerve is called:**

   a. Hiccough

   b. Wheeze

   c. Roar

   d. None of these

96. **An example of an anodyne expectorant is:**

   a. Codeine

   b. Ammonium chloride

   c. Potassium iodide

   d. Camphor

97. **Snoring respiration is characteristic of:**

   a. Pneumonia

   b. Heaves

   c. Paralysis of larynx

   d. Obstruction of the nasal passage

98. **The best site for auscultation of the heart is:**

   a. Space from 3rd to 6th rib on the left side

   b. Space from 3rd to 6th rib on the right side

   c. Space from 2nd to 5th rib on the left side

   d. Space from 2nd to 5th rib on the right side

99. **The groove present in the planum nasolabiale of horses is known as:**

   a. Philtrum

   b. Rugae

   c. Isthmus faucium

   d. None of these

100. **The instrument used for examination of the nasal passage is called a:**

   a. Rhino laryngoscope

   b. Cranio-graph

   c. Phonendoscope

   d. None of the above

101. **The process of tapping or striking the surface of the body using fingertips or an instrument is called:**

   a. Inspection

   b. Palpation

   c. Percussion

   d. Auscultation

102. **The instrument used for tapping or striking the surface of the body is called:**

   a. Stethoscope

   b. Pleximeter

c. Barometer

d. Phon-endoscope

103. **Shipping fever in cattle is caused by:**

a. *Pasteurella haemolytica*

b. *Pasteurella multocida*

c. *Mycoplasma mycoides*

d. *Chlamydia psittaci*

104. **The allergic test used for diagnosis of glanders is:**

a. Strauss reaction

b. Mallein test

c. Johnin test

d. Coggin's test

105. **A 'water-hammer pulse' is pathognomonic of:**

a. Interventricular septal defect

b. Patent ductus arteriosus

c. Dilated cardiomyopathy

d. Aortic incompetence

106. **Paper crackling rales on auscultation is suggestive of:**

a. Pneumonia

b. Bronchitis

c. Pulmonary emphysema

d. Pulmonary oedema

107. **Acute bovine pulmonary emphysema and oedema (ABPPE) is caused by:**

a. Excessive feeding of silage

b. Excessive feeding of lush greens

c. Feeding of mouldy hay

d. Excessive feeding of roughage

108. **Systolic and diastolic murmurs on auscultation is suggestive of:**

   a. Myocarditis

   b. Pericarditis

   c. Patent ductus arteriosus

   d. Vegetative endocarditis

109. **Diaphragmatic hernia is more common in:**

   a. Cows

   b. Buffalo

   c. Bullocks

   d. Sheep

110. **Persistent ruminal tympany, bradycardia and displaced heart sounds in cattle all suggest:**

   a. Traumatic pericarditis

   b. Traumatic reticulitis

   c. Diaphragmatic hernia

   d. Traumatic reticulo-peritonitis

111. **Which enzymes are important in apoptosis?**

   a. Caspases

   b. Lipases

   c. Aromatases

   d. Sulphydryl hydroxylases

112. **Conversion from less specialized cell types to more specialized cell types is called:**

   a. Dysplasia

   b. Metaplasia

   c. Anaplasia

   d. Hyperplasia

113. **Reed Sternberg cells are found in:**

    a. Hodgkin's disease

    b. Xanthomas

    c. Crigler-Najjar syndrome

    d. All of these

114. **Pneumonia caused by a parasite is known as:**

    a. Verminous pneumonia

    b. Bronchopneumonia

    c. Mycotic pneumonia

    d. All of these

115. **Dilatation of the bronchial lumen is called:**

    a. Atelectasis

    b. Bronchistenosis

    c. Bronchiectasis

    d. Emphysema

116. **Hypoxia:**

    a. Affects cells' aerobic respiration

    b. Affects cells' anaerobic respiration

    c. a and b

    d. Does not affect respiration

117. **Which statement is incorrect?**

    a. Ischaemia is a loss of blood supply due to obstructed blood flow

    b. In hypoxia glycolytic energy production can continue

    c. Ischaemia injures tissues faster than hypoxia

    d. Hypoxia injures tissues faster than ischaemia

118. **Myeloperoxidase-dependent killing is seen in:**

    a. Monocytes

    b. Neutrophils

    c. Basophils

    d. a and b

119. Strangles:

    a. Is a disease of younger animals

    b. Is a disease of older animals

    c. Is a disease of prepubertal animals

    d. Has no relation to age

120. Weibel-Palade bodies are found in:

    a. Platelets

    b. Leucocytes

    c. Endothelial cells

    d. a and c

121. Predisposing factors are also known as:

    a. Intrinsic or endogenous causes

    b. Extrinsic or exogenous causes

    c. a and b

    d. All of these

122. Phagocytic cells of the body are:

    a. Macrophages and lymphocytes

    b. Macrophages and neutrophils

    c. Neutrophils and lymphocytes

    d. Macrophages and plasma cells

123. L-selectins are present on:

    a. Platelets

    b. Leucocytes

    c. Endothelium

    d. All of these

124. **Modified macrophages in granuloma are called:**

    a. Goblet cells

    b. Giant cells

    c. Granulocytes

    d. Epithelioid cells

125. **An alteration that indicates the cause of a particular disease without doubt is called a:**

    a. Specific lesion

    b. Morbid lesion

    c. PM lesion

    d. Pathognomonic lesion

126. **Large granules of neutrophils are also known as:**

    a. Primary granules

    b. Azurophil granules

    c. Non-specific granules

    d. All of these

127. **Myeloperoxidase enzyme is present in:**

    a. Azurophil granules of neutrophils

    b. Specific granules of neutrophils

    c. Secondary granules of neutrophils

    d. Macrophages

128. **A common cause of infarction is:**

    a. Thrombi

    b. Emboli

    c. Hypoxia

    d. a and b

129. **Tuberculosis is an example of:**

    a. Coagulative necrosis

    b. Caseative necrosis

    c. Fat necrosis

    d. Liquefactive necrosis

130. Which is an example of liquefactive necrosis?

    a. White muscle disease

    b. Tuberculosis

    c. Abscess

    d. Adipose tissue trauma

131. A large quantity of hemosiderin is deposited in the liver and kidneys in:

    a. Babesiosis

    b. Leptospirosis

    c. Equine infectious anaemia

    d. Cyanide poisoning

132. 'Caisson disease' or 'bends' may lead to:

    a. Air emboli

    b. Fat emboli

    c. Septic emboli

    d. Thrombo emboli

133. Oedema fluid:

    a. Is non-inflammatory

    b. Is low in protein and other colloids

    c. Has specific gravity below 1.012

    d. All of these

134. The most common cause of cloudy swelling is:

    a. Hypoxia

    b. Alteration in the physical state of the protein

    c. Toxins

    d. None of these

135. **A 'ground glass' appearance of the cell cytoplasm is seen in:**

a. Cloudy swelling

b. Amyloid degeneration

c. Fatty change

d. All of these

136. **A common example of hyaline degeneration is:**

a. Zenker's degeneration of muscle

b. Equine azoturia

c. White muscle disease of calves

d. All of these

137. **An infarct is an area of:**

a. Hypoxia

b. Ischaemic necrosis

c. Haemorrhage

d. Gangrene

138. **Acute general active hyperaemia is observed in:**

a. Pasteurellosis

b. Swine erysipelas

c. Rabies

d. a and b

139. **Acute general passive hyperaemia is observed in:**

a. Pulmonary thrombosis and embolism

b. Hydropericardium, hemopericardium or pyopericardium

c. Sudden myocardial accidents

d. All of these

140. **Serum is rich in antienzyme in:**

a. Fowl

b. Hamsters

c. Guinea pigs

d. Rabbits

141. **Which statement is not true about avian inflammation?**

a. Chicken monocytes, basophils and thrombocytes are phagocytic

b. Eosinophils in chickens are not commonly found in allergic and parasitic inflammation

c. Giant cells are absent

d. Avian heterophil lacks myeloperoxidase

142. **A feature of viral inflammation is:**

a. Presence of lymphocytes

b. Presence of neutrophils

c. Suppuration

d. Granuloma formation

143. **Lysis of dead tissue by enzymes derived from inflammatory leucocytes is called:**

a. Autolysis

b. Chromatolysis

c. Heterolysis

d. None of these

144. **Which of these takes the form of small round cells of chronic inflammation?**

a. Lymphocytes and macrophages

b. Neutrophil and plasma cells

c. Macrophages and plasma cells

d. Lymphocytes and plasma cells

145. **Diffuse, flat and often irregular areas of bleeding are known as:**

a. Ecchymoses

b. Suffusions

    c. Extravasations

    d. Haemangiomas

146. The stages of cell injury are:

    a. Adaptation, reversible injury, irreversible injury and cell death

    b. Reversible injury, irreversible injury, adaptation and cell death

    c. Adaptation, irreversible injury and cell death

    d. Reversible injury, irreversible injury and cell death

147. 'Brisket disease' occurs because of:

    a. An increase in atmospheric pressure

    b. A decrease in atmospheric pressure

    c. Excess pressure on the heart

    d. All of these

148. The accumulation of excessive amounts of collagen in the form of raised tumorous scarring is known as:

    a. Keloid

    b. Proud flesh

    c. Exuberant granulation

    d. All of these

149. Fragmentation of the nucleus in a cell is known as:

    a. Pyknosis

    b. Karyorrhexis

    c. Karyolysis

    d. Chromatolysis

150. The 'first line of cellular defence' in inflammation is:

    a. Monocytes

    b. Macrophages

    c. Lymphocytes

    d. Neutrophils

151. **Escape of RBC from intact blood vessels is known as:**

 a. Diapedesis

 b. Rhexis

 c. Ecchymoses

 d. Extravasation

152. **Caisson disease or decompression sickness occurs because of:**

 a. Increase in atmospheric pressure

 b. Decrease in atmospheric pressure

 c. Excess pressure on the heart

 d. All of these

153. **Hydropic degeneration is closely related to:**

 a. Hyaline degeneration

 b. Cloudy swelling

 c. Mucous degeneration

 d. Amyloid degeneration

154. **Infiltration of the pleomorphic lymphoid cells is seen in:**

 a. Lymphoid leukosis

 b. Marek's disease

 c. IBH

 d. Newcastle disease

155. **The disease caused by influenza virus type-A subtype H5N1 is known as:**

 a. Swine flu

 b. Equine influenza

 c. Bird flu

 d. Human flu

156. **A vertically transmitted bacterial disease of poultry is:**

 a. Pullorum disease and fowl typhoid

 b. Chronic respiratory disease

c. Colibacillosis

d. All of these

157. Allergic inflammation is characterized by:

a. Lymphocytes

b. Monocytes

c. Neutrophils

d. Eosinophils

158. Infarct is an example of:

a. Coagulative necrosis

b. Liquefactive necrosis

c. Caseative necrosis

d. Fat necrosis

159. The 'second line of cellular defence' is:

a. Neutrophils

b. Plasma cells

c. Macrophages

d. Giant cells

160. Which type of inflammation is seen in tuberculosis?

a. Fibrinous

b. Haemorrhagic

c. Granulomatous

d. Suppurative

161. An example of a foreign-body giant cell is:

a. Langhan's giant cell of tuberculosis

b. Giant cell of Johne's disease

c. Giant cell of actinomycosis and blastomycosis

d. All of these

162. **Which giant cells have a characteristic ring of nuclei at the periphery?**

    a. Touton giant cells of xanthomas

    b. Langhan's giant cells of TB

    c. Reed-Sternberg cells of Hodgkin's disease

    d. Tumour giant cells

163. **Which vitamin plays an important role in wound healing?**

    a. Vitamin A

    b. Vitamin C

    c. Vitamin D

    d. Vitamin K

164. **Drugs such as penicillin interfere with wound healing by:**

    a. Preventing synthesis of hyaluronic acid

    b. Preventing collagen cross linking

    c. Preventing angiogenesis

    d. Preventing protein synthesis

165. **Which chemical mediator of inflammation is known as 'endogenous pyrogen'?**

    a. $PGF_{2\alpha}$

    b. PGG_2

    c. PGE_2

    d. PGI_2

166. **The colloidal carbon technique is used in the identification of:**

    a. Anthracosis in the liver

    b. Anthracosis in the lungs

    c. Leaking vessels in inflammation

    d. None of these

167. **The first line of defence in tumour and viral infections is:**
    a. Macrophage
    b. Neutrophil
    c. NK cell
    d. None of these

168. **Blue babies' condition is due to:**
    a. Stenosis of pulmonary valves
    b. Patent foramen ovale
    c. Interventricular septal defects
    d. All of these

169. **Perivascular lymphocytic infiltration just outside the blood vessel is known as:**
    a. Perivascular cuffing
    b. Satellitosis
    c. Gitter cells
    d. Plasma cells

170. **Fowl typhoid is caused by:**
    a. *Salmonella pullorum*
    b. *Salmonella gallinarum*
    c. *Salmonella typhimurium*
    d. *Salmonella typhosa*

171. **Deposition of calcium carbonate or calcium dust in the lungs is known as:**
    a. Acanthosis
    b. Chalicosis
    c. Anthracosis
    d. Argyrosis

172. 'Biphasic fever' or 'diphasic fever' is characteristic of :

a. Rabies

b. Canine distemper

c. Infectious canine hepatitis

d. Bovine ephemeral fever

173. **Extensive demyelination of the neurons occurs in:**

a. Canine distemper

b. Infectious canine hepatitis

c. Leptospirosis

d. Rabies

174. **'Sulfur granules' in yellowish pus is seen in:**

a. Glanders

b. Strangles

c. Staphylococcosis

d. Actinomycosis

175. **'Chattering' in mice is due to:**

a. *Clostridium piliformis*

b. *Klebsiella pneumoniae*

c. *Citrobacter rodentium*

d. *Mycoplasma pulmonis*

176. **Orf is mainly a disease of:**

a. Cattle

b. Swine

c. Horses

d. Sheep and goats

177. **A common site for the primary tumour in metastasis is the:**

a. Lungs

b. Liver

    c. Intestine

    d. Brain

178. **Accumulation of air in pericardium is called:**

    a. Pneumothorax

    b. Pneumopericardium

    c. Pyopericardium

    d. Hydropericardium

179. **Failure of the alveoli to open and contain air is known as:**

    a. Atelectasis

    b. Bronchistenosis

    c. Bronchiectasis

    d. Emphysema

180. **Which of these is not a true aneurysm?**

    a. Fusiform

    b. Cirsoid

    c. Dissecting

    d. Arteriovenous

181. **In which stage of pneumonia can fibrin be clearly seen?**

    a. Stage of resolution

    b. Stage of red hepatization

    c. Stage of grey hepatization

    d. Stage of congestion

182. **The sparer of Vitamin A is:**

    a. Vitamin A

    b. Vitamin K

    c. Vitamin D

    d. Vitamin E

183. **The most common form of IB in poultry is:**

    a. Respiratory

    b. Reproductive

    c. Nephritic

    d. None of these

184. **Subcutaneous oedema of the face (swollen face) and wattles, together with conjunctivitis is seen in:**

    a. Pullorum disease

    b. Fowl cholera

    c. Infectious coryza

    d. Fowl typhoid

185. **Infectious coryza is caused by:**

    a. *Haemophilus paragallinarum*

    b. *Pasteurella multocida*

    c. *Mycoplasma gallisepticum*

    d. *Aspergillus fumigatous*

186. **Fowl cholera is caused by:**

    a. *Haemophilus paragallinarum*

    b. *Pasteurella multocida*

    c. *Mycoplasma gallisepticum*

    d. *Aspergillus fumigatous*

187. **Gapes is a characteristic feature of:**

    a. *Trachealis bronchi*

    b. *Heterakis galli*

    c. *Syngamus trachea*

    d. *Trachealis pulmoni*

188. **Caseous air sacculitis is observed in:**

    a. Infectious coryza

    b. Chronic respiratory disease

    c. Avian chlamydiosis

    d. Fowl spirochaetosis

189. **Defective oxygenation of the blood in the pulmonary circuit is known as:**

    a. Stagnant anoxia

    b. Anaemic anoxia

    c. Anoxic anoxia

    d. Histotoxic anoxia

190. **A vertically transmitted disease in poultry is:**

    a. Chronic respiratory disease

    b. Avian encephalomyelitis

    c. Chicken infectious anaemia

    d. All of these

191. **Which of these is a zoonotic disease?**

    a. Avian TB

    b. Fowl paratyphoid

    c. Campylobacteriosis

    d. All of these

192. **Marek's disease is caused by:**

    a. Gallid Herpesvirus 1

    b. Birnavirus

    c. Gallid Herpesvirus 2

    d. Circovirus

193.   Infectious laryngotracheitis is caused by:

a. Gallid Herpesvirus - 1

b. Birnavirus

c. Gallid Herpesvirus - 2

d. Circovirus

194.   Brooder pneumonia is caused by:

a. *Aspergillus fumigatus*

b. *Aspergillus flavus*

c. *Mycoplasma gallisepticum*

d. a and b

195.   Presence of cheesy deposits in the air sacs is indicative of:

a. Infectious coryza

b. Chronic respiratory disease

c. Avian chlamydiosis

d. Fowl spirochaetosis

196.   Death of birds after paralytic symptoms in very cloudy rainy seasons with high humidity, poor ventilation and overcrowding is indicative of:

a. Carbon monoxide poisoning

b. Colibacillosis

c. Heat stroke

d. Smothering

197.   Avian influenza or bird flu is caused by:

a. Orthomyxovirus

b. Paramyxovirus

c. Retrovirus

d. Rhabdovirus

198. **Mucopurulent exudates in the nares, fibrinopurulent exudates over the pericardium, pleura, air sacs, hepatomegaly, marked enlargement of spleen and necrotic foci on its surface are observed in:**

   a. Avian influenza

   b. Infectious bronchitis

   c. Ranikhet disease

   d. Mycoplasmosis

199. **Infectious bronchitis is caused by:**

   a. Retrovirus

   b. Enterovirus

   c. Circovirus

   d. Coronavirus

200. **Intranuclear inclusion bodies in the tracheal epithelium is characteristic of:**

   a. Ranikhet disease

   b. Infectious bronchitis

   c. Infectious bursal disease

   d. Infectious laryngotracheitis

201. **Psittacosis is mainly a disease of:**

   a. Elephants

   b. Birds

   c. Horses

   d. Sheep

202. **A characteristic lesion of chicken infectious anaemia is:**

   a. Thymic atrophy

   b. Bone marrow atrophy

   c. Bone marrow aplasia

   d. All of these

203. **Swelling of the infraorbital sinus with cheesy exudate is seen in:**

    a. Chronic respiratory disease

    b. Colibacillosis

    c. Infectious bursal disease

    d. Infectious coryza

204. **Tularaemia in rabbits is caused by:**

    a. *Francisella tularensis*

    b. *Moraxella muris*

    c. *Pasteurella piliformis*

    d. *Citrobacter muris*

205. **Infectious bursal disease virus destroys:**

    a. B-cells

    b. T-cells

    c. Heterophils

    d. Macrophages

206. **The causal agent of CBPP is:**

    a. *Mycoplasma mycoides* subsp. *mycoides*

    b. *Mycoplasma mycoides* subsp. *capri*

    c. *Mycoplasma agalactiae*

    d. *Mycoplasma gallisepticum*

207. **The causal agent of Peste des petits in ruminants is:**

    a. Birnavirus

    b. Herpesvirus

    c. Morbillivirus

    d. Orbivirus

208. **Pseudo tuberculosis is caused by:**

    a. *Mycobacterium tuberculosis*

    b. *Yersinia pseudotuberculosis*

c. *Mycobacterium leprae*

d. *Corynebacterium pseudotuberculosis*

209. **Kennel cough in dogs is caused by:**

a. *Streptococcus pneumonia*

b. *Bordetella avium*

c. *Streptococcus zooepidemicus*

d. *Bordetella bronchiseptica*

210. **For diagnosis of avian Influenza in chickens, inoculation is done by which method?**

a. Oral route

b. Aerosol route

c. IV

d. IM

211. **Tropical pulmonary eosinophilia is mainly seen due to:**

a. Cercarial reaction

b. Nematode larvae

c. Arthropods

d. Pollen allergy

212. **Lungworm vaccine for cattle was commercially introduced by Jarret and co-workers in:**

a. 1972

b. 1959

c. 1960

d. 1872

213. **The trematode parasite found in pairs in the lungs is:**

a. *Dicrocoelium* spp.

b. *Paragonimus* spp.

c. *Opisthorchis* spp.

d. *Schistosoma* spp.

214. **The parasite found in the lung tissue of wild felines is:**

   a. *Paragoni muskelicotii*

   b. *Bivitello bilharzianairi*

   c. *Protofasciola robusta*

   d. *Fasciola jacksoni*

215. **The tracheal worm in poultry is:**

   a. *Heterakis gallinarum*

   b. *Ascaridia galli*

   c. *Syngamus trachea*

   d. *Prosthogonimus ovatus*

216. **Parasitic catarrhal bronchitis in sheep is caused by:**

   a. *Dictyocaulus viviparus*

   b. *Dictyocaulus arnfieldi*

   c. *Metastrongylus apri*

   d. *Dictyocaulus filaria*

217. **Husk/hoose in cattle is caused by:**

   a. *Dictyocaulus viviparus*

   b. *Dictyocaulus filaria*

   c. *Dictyocaulus arnfieldi*

   d. *Dictyocaulus cameli*

218. **Lungworm in cats is:**

   a. *Aelurostrongylus abstrusus*

   b. *Filaroides osleri*

   c. *Oslerus osleri*

   d. *Filaroides hirthi*

219. **The lungworm infecting rats is:**

   a. *Angiostrongylus cantonensis*

   b. *Protostrongylus rufescence*

c. *Metastrongylus salmi*

d. None of these

220. Laboured breathing or gape is characteristic of:

a. Avian influenza

b. Histomoniasis

c. Syngamiasis

d. Fowl pox

221. A common lungworm in equines is:

a. *Dictyocaulus viviparus*

b. *Capillaria aerophila*

c. *Muellerius capillaris*

d. *Dictyocaulus arnfieldi*

222. Hourglass-shaped pharynx is observed in:

a. *Oxyspirura mansoni*

b. *Oxyuris equi*

c. *Heterakis gallinarum*

d. *Contracaecum*

223. Funnel-shaped pharynx is observed in:

a. *Habronema majus*

b. *Habronema microstoma*

c. *Draschia megastoma*

d. *Habronema muscae*

224. Which lungworm is seen in dogs?

a. *Filaroides osleri*

b. *Oslerus osleri*

c. *Filaroides hirthi*

d. All of these

225. **Which parasite is responsible for forming nodules in the lungs of cats?**

a. *Aelurostrongylus abstrusus*

b. *Filaroides osleri*

c. *Oslerus osleri*

d. *Filaroides hirthi*

226. **Lungworm larvae with a short 'S'-shaped tail are:**

a. *Aelurostrongylus abstrusus*

b. *Filaroides hirthi*

c. *Filaroides osleri*

d. *Angistrongylus vasorum*

227. **Lungworm L1 larvae with a small cuticular knob at anterior extremity and numerous brown food granules in the intestinal cells are:**

a. *Filaroides osleri*

b. *Dictyocaulus filaria*

c. *Dictyocaulus viviparus*

d. *Angistrongylus vasorum*

228. **Which lungworm larvae are disseminated by *Pilobolus* fungus?**

a. *Filaroides osleri*

b. *Dictyocaulus filaria*

c. *Dictyocaulus viviparus*

d. *Angistrongylus vasorum*

229. **Nodular lungworm of sheep and goat is:**

a. *Cystocaulus nigrescens*

b. *Protostrongylus rufescens*

c. *Muellerius capillaris*

d. All of these

230. **Donkey lungworm is:**

   a. *Dictyocaulus viviparus*

   b. *Dictyocaulus filaria*

   c. *Dictyocaulus arnfieldi*

   d. *Dictyocaulus cameli*

231. **The name for lungworm in which swelling in the female tail covers the vulva and anus is:**

   a. *Dictyocaulus*

   b. *Protostrongylus*

   c. *Metastrongylus*

   d. *Muellerius*

232. **Which lungworm have broad membranous cuticular expansions in the spicule?**

   a. *Dictyocaulus*

   b. *Protostrongylus*

   c. *Metastrongylus*

   d. *Muellerius*

233. **What is the name for lungworm L1 spineless larvae with a wavy outline to the tip of the tail?**

   a. *Cystocaulus nigrescens*

   b. *Protostrongylus rufescens*

   c. *Muellerius capillaris*

   d. All of these

234. **Lobular pneumonia in sheep is caused by:**

   a. *Cystocaulus nigrescens*

   b. *Protostrongylus rufescens*

   c. *Muellerius capillaris*

   d. All of these

235. **Which parasite is thought to be involved in the transmission of swine influenza/swine fever virus?**

    a. *Stephanurus dentatus*

    b. *Oesophagostomum*

    c. *Metastrongylus*

    d. *Macracanthorhynchus*

236. **Red lungworm in sheep and goat is:**

    a. *Cystocaulus nigrescens*

    b. *Protostrongylus rufescens*

    c. *Muellerius capillaris*

    d. All of these

237. **Which parasite is found in the trachea of birds?**

    a. *Syngamus trachea*

    b. *Cyathostoma bronchialis*

    c. *Cyathostoma variegatum*

    d. All of these

238. **A parasitic nematode found in the trachea, bronchi, nasal cavity and frontal sinus of dogs and foxes is likely to be:**

    a. *Capillaria bovis*

    b. *Capillaria caudinflata*

    c. *Capillaria aerophila*

    d. *Capillaria philippinensis*

239. **A 3-year-old dog presented with progressive weight loss, pneumonia and tubular regurgitation immediately after food intake is a good candidate for:**

    a. Congenital megaoesophagus

    b. Acquired megaoesophagus

    c. Ranula

    d. Choke

240. **Haemorrhagic mixed exudate originating from the lungs is known as:**

a. Epistaxix

b. Hemoptysis

c. Hematemesis

d. All of these

241. **For an asthmatic feline patient, all of the following are indicated except:**

a. Oxygen therapy

b. Dexamethasone

c. Aminophylline

d. Ketoprofen

242. **Histotoxic anoxia develops in:**

a. Rape and kale poisoning

b. Cyanide poisoning

c. Urget poisoning

d. All of these

243. **Which is an example of an inhalant expectorant?**

a. TT oil

b. Belladonna

c. Codeine

d. Creoline

244. **Ammonium chloride is a:**

a. Saline expectorant

b. Stimulant expectorant

c. Inhalant expectorant

d. Bronchodilator

245. Which disease of poultry is not transmitted vertically?

a. Avian encephalomyelitis

b. Pullorum disease

c. Egg drops syndrome

d. Marek's disease

246. Purulent exudate in the pleural cavity, caused by pyogenic bacteria or fungi reaching the thoracic cavity is known as:

a. Empyema

b. Hemothorax

c. Chylothorax

d. Pneumothorax

247. Accumulation of air in the pleural cavity is known as:

a. Empyema

b. Hemothorax

c. Chylothorax

d. Pneumothorax

248. Accumulation of chyle in the pleural cavity is known as:

a. Empyema

b. Hemothorax

c. Chylothorax

d. Pneumothorax

249. Chronic pneumonia, characterized by firm diffuse lesions due to hyperplasia of the lymphoid follicles, hyperplasia of smooth muscle around bronchioles, diffuse fibrosis and diffuse lymphocytic infiltration, in sheep is called:

a. Maedi

b. Sheep flu

c. Chylothorax

d. PPR

250. **Pulmonary oedema is a characteristic sign of:**

 a. PCF

 b. LHF

 c. RHF

 d. Pneumonia

Answers

1.	b	31.	a	61.	c	91.	a
2.	b	32.	a	62.	d	92.	c
3.	a	33.	a	63.	a	93.	b
4.	d	34.	b	64.	a	94.	d
5.	c	35.	c	65.	c	95.	a
6.	a	36.	a	66.	b	96.	a
7.	a	37.	d	67.	a	97.	d
8.	a	38.	d	68.	c	98.	c
9.	c	39.	a	69.	c	99.	a
10.	d	40.	c	70.	a	100.	a
11.	b	41.	b	71.	b	101.	c
12.	b	42.	a	72.	c	102.	b
13.	d	43.	c	73.	d	103.	a
14.	b	44.	a	74.	d	104.	b
15.	d	45.	d	75.	a	105.	d
16.	c	46.	b	76.	c	106.	c
17.	d	47.	d	77.	b	107.	b
18.	a	48.	b	78.	b	108.	c
19.	c	49.	b	79.	a	109.	b
20.	a	50.	a	80.	a	110.	c
21.	a	51.	a	81.	c	111.	a
22.	a	52.	a	82.	b	112.	b
23.	d	53.	d	83.	d	113.	a
24.	a	54.	c	84.	d	114.	a
25.	a	55.	c	85.	b	115.	c
26.	c	56.	d	86.	d	116.	a
27.	a	57.	d	87.	d	117.	d
28.	a	58.	d	88.	b	118.	d
29.	a	59.	a	89.	d	119.	a
30.	c	60.	a	90.	a	120.	c

(Continued)

121.	a	154.	b	187.	c	220.	c
122.	b	155.	c	188.	b	221.	d
123.	b	156.	d	189.	a	222.	a
124.	d	157.	d	190.	d	223.	c
125.	d	158.	a	191.	d	224.	d
126.	d	159.	c	192.	c	225.	a
127.	a	160.	c	193.	a	226.	c
128.	d	161.	d	194.	d	227.	b
129.	b	162.	a	195.	b	228.	c
130.	c	163.	b	196.	d	229.	a
131.	c	164.	b	197.	a	230.	c
132.	a	165.	c	198.	d	231.	c
133.	d	166.	c	199.	d	232.	b
134.	a	167.	c	200.	d	233.	b
135.	a	168.	d	201.	b	234.	b
136.	d	169.	a	202.	d	235.	c
137.	b	170.	b	203.	d	236.	b
138.	d	171.	b	204.	a	237.	d
139.	d	172.	b	205.	a	238.	c
140.	d	173.	a	206.	a	239.	b
141.	c	174.	d	207.	c	240.	b
142.	a	175.	d	208.	b	241.	d
143.	c	176.	d	209.	d	242.	b
144.	d	177.	a	210.	b	243.	a
145.	b	178.	b	211.	b	244.	a
146.	a	179.	a	212.	b	245.	d
147.	b	180.	c	213.	b	246.	a
148.	a	181.	c	214.	a	247.	d
149.	b	182.	d	215.	c	248.	c
150.	d	183.	a	216.	d	249.	a
151.	a	184.	c	217.	a	250.	b
152.	a	185.	a	218.	a		
153.	b	186.	b	219.	a		

5 Diseases of the Endocrine System

K.S. Prasanna

Introduction

The endocrine system is one of the major systems in the body that controls almost all the metabolic functions. It consists of the pituitary, pancreas, adrenal, thyroid and parathyroid glands, and the reproductive organs testes and ovaries. Hormones are directly released into the blood and any kind of malfunction in any of these organs leads to a series of pathological conditions. The general disease conditions are congenital abnormalities, infectious and inflammatory conditions, autoimmune reactions and deficiency conditions. The 'master gland', the pituitary, produces the stimulating or inhibiting hormones which act on the other endocrine glands. The release of hormones from the pituitary is regulated by the hormones from the hypothalamus region of the brain.

© CAB International 2024. *Key Questions in Clinical Farm Animal Medicine Volume 1: Principles of Disease Examination, Diagnosis and Management* (ed. T. Rana) DOI: 10.1079/9781800624788.0005

Multiple Choice Questions

1. **Which of the glands have a major role in regulating sodium and potassium levels in the body?**

   a. Thyroid

   b. Adrenal

   c. Pituitary

   d. Liver

2. **What is the main function of the thyroid gland?**

   a. To regulate blood glucose levels

   b. To regulate body temperature and metabolism

   c. To regulate blood calcium levels

   d. To regulate blood pressure

3. **Which hormone is primarily secreted by the thyroid gland in animals?**

   a. Insulin

   b. Oestrogen

   c. Thyroxine

   d. Testosterone

4. **What is the effect of hyperthyroidism in animals?**

   a. Weight gain

   b. Lethargy

   c. Increased heart rate

   d. Hypertension

5. **Which of the following can cause hypothyroidism in animals?**

   a. Overactive thyroid gland

   b. Autoimmune disease

   c. Excessive iodine intake

   d. None of these

6. **Which of the following is a common symptom of hypothyroidism in dogs?**

   a. Increased appetite

   b. Weight gain

   c. Hyperactivity

   d. Aggressiveness

7. **Which of the following animals is prone to goitre due to iodine deficiency?**

   a. Cows

   b. Horses

   c. Sheep

   d. Dogs

8. **What is the role of iodine in the thyroid gland of animals?**

   a. To regulate blood glucose levels

   b. To regulate body temperature and metabolism

   c. To regulate blood calcium levels

   d. To synthesize thyroid hormones

9. **The pituitary gland is often referred to as the master gland because it secretes hormones that:**

   a. Control other endocrine glands

   b. Regulates body temperature

   c. Regulates blood glucose levels

   d. Regulates heart rate

10. **Which of the following hormones is secreted by the anterior pituitary gland?**

    a. Oxytocin

    b. Vasopressin

    c. Prolactin

    d. Adrenocorticotropic hormone (ACTH)

11. **Which hormone is responsible for stimulating milk production in lactating animals?**

   a. Oxytocin

   b. Growth hormone

   c. Thyroid-stimulating hormone (TSH)

   d. Prolactin

12. **The posterior pituitary gland secretes which of the following hormones?**

   a. Luteinizing hormone (LH)

   b. Follicle-stimulating hormone (FSH)

   c. Oxytocin

   d. Prolactin

13. **What is the function of adrenocorticotropic hormone (ACTH)?**

   a. To stimulate the adrenal glands to release cortisol

   b. To stimulate the thyroid gland to release thyroid hormones

   c. To stimulate the pancreas to release insulin

   d. To stimulate the liver to produce glucose

14. **Which of the following conditions is caused by overproduction of growth hormones in animals?**

   a. Gigantism

   b. Dwarfism

   c. Hypothyroidism

   d. Hyperthyroidism

15. **In which part of the reproductive tract does fertilization typically occur in female animals?**

   a. Ovary

   b. Oviduct

   c. Uterus

   d. Vagina

16. **Which of the following hormones is primarily responsible for the development of secondary sex characteristics in female animals?**

    a. Oestrogen

    b. Progesterone

    c. Luteinizing hormone (LH)

    d. Follicle-stimulating hormone (FSH)

17. **Which of the following structures produces progesterone in the ovary?**

    a. Corpus luteum

    b. Ovarian follicle

    c. Oviduct

    d. Uterus

18. **Which of the following is a condition in which the ovary twists around its own axis, disrupting blood flow to the organ?**

    a. Ovarian cyst

    b. Ovarian cancer

    c. Ovarian torsion

    d. Polycystic ovary syndrome (PCOS)

19. **Which of the following hormones is responsible for the development and maturation of ovarian follicles?**

    a. Oestrogen

    b. Progesterone

    c. Luteinizing hormone (LH)

    d. Follicle-stimulating hormone (FSH)

20. **Which of the following is a common reproductive disorder in male animals characterized by the accumulation of fluid in the scrotum?**

    a. Testicular torsion

    b. Epididymitis

c. Hydrocele

d. Varicocele

21. **Which of the following accessory glands produces a fluid that helps to neutralize the acidic environment of the female reproductive tract?**

a. Cowper's gland

b. Prostate gland

c. Seminal vesicles

d. Bulbourethral gland

22. **Which of the following hormones is responsible for the development of secondary sex characteristics in male animals?**

a. Oestrogen

b. Progesterone

c. Luteinizing hormone (LH)

d. Testosterone

23. **Which of the following structures is responsible for the storage and maturation of sperm in male animals?**

a. Testis

b. Epididymis

c. Vas deferens

d. Urethra

24. **Which of the following accessory glands produces a fluid that helps to lubricate the urethra during ejaculation?**

a. Cowper's gland

b. Prostate gland

c. Seminal vesicles

d. Bulbourethral gland

25. **Which of the following is a condition in which the testis twists around its own axis, disrupting blood flow to the organ?**

    a. Testicular torsion

    b. Epididymitis

    c. Hydrocele

    d. Varicocele

26. **How many parathyroid glands are typically present in cats?**

    a. 1

    b. 2

    c. 3

    d. 4

27. **Which of the following hormones is produced by the parathyroid gland?**

    a. Thyroxine

    b. Insulin

    c. Glucagon

    d. Parathyroid hormone (PTH)

28. **What is the primary function of parathyroid hormone (PTH)?**

    a. To increase calcium levels in the blood

    b. To decrease calcium levels in the blood

    c. To increase glucose levels in the blood

    d. To decrease glucose levels in the blood

29. **What effect does PTH have on bone tissue?**

    a. It increases bone formation

    b. It decreases bone formation

    c. It increases bone resorption

    d. It decreases bone resorption

30. **What is the name of the condition that results from overproduction of PTH?**

   a. Hyperthyroidism

   b. Hypothyroidism

   c. Hyperparathyroidism

   d. Hypoparathyroidism

31. **What are the two main regions of the adrenal gland?**

   a. Cortex and medulla

   b. Anterior and posterior

   c. Superior and inferior

   d. Left and right

32. **What type of hormone is primarily produced by the adrenal cortex?**

   a. Cortisol

   b. Adrenaline

   c. Noradrenaline

   d. Epinephrine

33. **What effect does cortisol have on the body?**

   a. It increases blood pressure

   b. It decreases blood pressure

   c. It increases blood glucose levels

   d. It decreases blood glucose levels

34. **What is the primary function of the adrenal medulla?**

   a. To produce cortisol

   b. To produce adrenaline and noradrenaline

   c. To regulate blood pressure

   d. To regulate blood glucose levels

35. **What is the name of the condition that results from overpro-duction of cortisol?**

   a. Cushing's syndrome

   b. Addison's disease

   c. Diabetes insipidus

   d. Hyperthyroidism

36. **Vasopressin is a hormone released from:**

   a. Adrenal

   b. Pituitary

   c. Thyroid

   d. Testis

37. **What is the main function of the pancreas in animals?**

   a. To produce insulin

   b. To produce glucagon

   c. To produce digestive enzymes

   d. To regulate blood pressure

38. **The anterior pituitary is derived from the oropharyngeal ectoderm of:**

   a. Rathkei's pouch

   b. Glisson's pouch

   c. Pars nervosa

   d. Rathkei's notch

39. **Which hormone is primarily produced by beta cells in the pancreas?**

   a. Insulin

   b. Glucagon

   c. Somatostatin

   d. Amylin

40. **What is the name of the condition that results from a deficiency in insulin production?**

   a. Type 1 diabetes

   b. Type 2 diabetes

   c. Hypoglycaemia

   d. Hyperglycaemia

41. **What is the name of the condition that results from resistance to insulin?**

   a. Type 1 diabetes

   b. Type 2 diabetes

   c. Hypoglycaemia

   d. Hyperglycaemia

42. **What is the name of the hormone that is co-secreted with insulin by beta cells?**

   a. Glucagon

   b. Somatostatin

   c. Amylin

   d. Adrenaline

43. **What is the function of somatostatin in the pancreas?**

   a. To stimulate insulin production

   b. To inhibit insulin production

   c. To stimulate glucagon production

   d. To inhibit glucagon production

44. **Which of the following hormones is not produced by the hypothalamus gland?**

   a. Thyrotropin-releasing hormone (TRH)

   b. Gonadotropin-releasing hormone (GnRH)

   c. Adrenocorticotropic hormone (ACTH)

   d. Growth hormone-releasing hormone (GHRH)

45. **What is the main function of the hypothalamus gland?**

    a. To regulate body temperature

    b. To produce hormones that control other glands

    c. To produce digestive enzymes

    d. To regulate muscle movement

46. **What are the two main types of cells found in the pancreas?**

    a. Alpha and beta

    b. Red and white

    c. Neurons and glial

    d. Epithelial and muscle

47. **Which hormone does the hypothalamus release to stimulate the release of growth hormone from the pituitary gland?**

    a. Thyrotropin-releasing hormone (TRH)

    b. Gonadotropin-releasing hormone (GnRH)

    c. Adrenocorticotropic hormone (ACTH)

    d. Growth hormone-releasing hormone (GHRH)

48. **Which of the following is not a role of melatonin in animals?**

    a. Regulating sleep patterns

    b. Regulating the timing of seasonal breeding

    c. Regulating body temperature

    d. Stimulating muscle growth

49. **Which of the hormones from the hypothalamus influence the release of follicle-stimulating hormone (FSH) and luteinizing hormone (LH) from the pituitary gland?**

    a. Thyrotropin-releasing hormone (TRH)

    b. Gonadotropin-releasing hormone (GnRH)

    c. Adrenocorticotropic hormone (ACTH)

    d. Growth hormone-releasing hormone (GHRH)

50. **What is the function of the hormone oxytocin, which is produced in the hypothalamus?**

   a. To stimulate uterine contractions during childbirth

   b. To stimulate milk production in the mammary glands

   c. To regulate body temperature

   d. To stimulate muscle movement

51. **What is the function of the hormone vasopressin, which is produced in the hypothalamus?**

   a. To stimulate uterine contractions during childbirth

   b. To stimulate milk production in the mammary glands

   c. To regulate body temperature

   d. To regulate water balance in the body

52. **Which of the following is a symptom of hyperparathyroidism?**

   a. Low blood pressure

   b. Fatigue

   c. Muscle weakness

   d. Weight gain

53. **Which of these is a type of tumour originating in the adrenal medulla?**

   a. Medullary blastoma

   b. Medullary carcinoma

   c. Pheochromocytoma

   d. Chromaffinoma

54. **What is the treatment for hyperparathyroidism?**

   a. Surgery to remove the affected gland

   b. Medications to decrease PTH production

   c. Radiation therapy to the parathyroid gland

   d. Lifestyle changes to decrease calcium intake

55. **Which of the chemicals can induce hypothyroidism in pigs?**

    a. Urea

    b. Thiourea

    c. Monosodium glutamate

    d. Glutathione

56. **How many adrenal glands are present in most animals?**

    a. 1

    b. 2

    c. 3

    d. 4

57. **What is the primary function of the testis in male animals?**

    a. To produce testosterone

    b. To produce sperm

    c. To produce oestrogen

    d. To produce progesterone

58. **Which hormone is responsible for stimulating the production of testosterone in male animals?**

    a. Oestrogen

    b. Progesterone

    c. Luteinizing hormone (LH)

    d. Follicle-stimulating hormone (FSH)

59. **Which of the following accessory glands produces the majority of the fluid that makes up semen?**

    a. Cowper's gland

    b. Prostate gland

    c. Seminal vesicles

    d. Bulbourethral gland

60.   **Which of the following hormones is responsible for regulating the production of sperm in male animals?**

   a. Oestrogen

   b. Progesterone

   c. Luteinizing hormone (LH)

   d. Follicle-stimulating hormone (FSH)

61.   **Which of the following structures produces oestrogen in the ovary?**

   a. Corpus luteum

   b. Ovarian follicle

   c. Oviduct

   d. Uterus

62.   **Which of the following hormones is responsible for maintaining pregnancy in female animals?**

   a. Oestrogen

   b. Progesterone

   c. Luteinizing hormone (LH)

   d. Follicle-stimulating hormone (FSH)

63.   **Which of the following is a reproductive disorder in pigs characterized by cysts on the ovaries?**

   a. Endometriosis

   b. Polycystic ovary syndrome (PCOS)

   c. Ovarian cancer

   d. Uterine fibroids

64.   **Which of the following conditions is caused by a deficiency in antidiuretic hormone (ADH), which is produced in the hypothalamus?**

   a. Diabetes insipidus

   b. Diabetes mellitus

   c. Cushing's syndrome

   d. Acromegaly

65. **Which of the following hormones is not regulated by the hypothalamus?**

    a. Thyroid-stimulating hormone (TSH)

    b. Adrenocorticotropic hormone (ACTH)

    c. Follicle-stimulating hormone (FSH)

    d. Insulin

66. **What is the name of the hormone produced by the pineal gland that regulates the timing of seasonal breeding in animals?**

    a. Melatonin

    b. Progesterone

    c. Oestrogen

    d. Testosterone

67. **What is the role of melatonin in regulating the timing of seasonal breeding?**

    a. It stimulates the release of reproductive hormones

    b. It inhibits the release of reproductive hormones

    c. It directly stimulates ovulation

    d. It has no effect on reproductive hormones

68. **Which of the following animals has the highest levels of melatonin production?**

    a. Nocturnal animals

    b. Diurnal animals

    c. Animals that hibernate

    d. Aquatic animals

69. **What is the primary hormone produced by the pineal gland?**

    a. Melatonin

    b. Thyroxine

    c. Epinephrine

    d. Glucagon

70. **What is the main function of melatonin?**

    a. To regulate the sleep-wake cycle

    b. To stimulate muscle movement

    c. To regulate blood glucose levels

    d. To stimulate the adrenal glands

71. **What stimulates the release of melatonin from the pineal gland?**

    a. Sunlight

    b. Darkness

    c. High levels of stress

    d. Exercise

72. **What is the function of calcitonin in relation to the parathyroid gland?**

    a. It stimulates the release of PTH

    b. It inhibits the release of PTH

    c. It has no effect on PTH

    d. It blocks the action of PTH

73. **Which of the following minerals is regulated by PTH?**

    a. Sodium

    b. Chloride

    c. Calcium

    d. Potassium

74. **What effect does adrenaline have on the body?**

    a. It increases heart rate and blood pressure

    b. It decreases heart rate and blood pressure

    c. It decreases blood glucose levels

    d. It increases blood glucose levels

75. **What effect does noradrenaline have on the body?**

   a. It increases heart rate and blood pressure

   b. It decreases heart rate and blood pressure

   c. It decreases blood glucose levels

   d. It increases blood glucose levels

76. **Which of the following is a symptom of adrenal insufficiency?**

   a. High blood pressure

   b. Low blood pressure

   c. High blood glucose levels

   d. Low blood glucose levels

77. **Which hormone does the hypothalamus release to inhibit the release of prolactin from the pituitary gland?**

   a. Prolactin-releasing hormone (PRH)

   b. Prolactin-inhibiting hormone (PIH)

   c. Luteinizing hormone-releasing hormone (LHRH)

   d. Follicle-stimulating hormone-releasing hormone (FSHRH)

78. **Which hormone does the hypothalamus release to stimulate the release of follicle-stimulating hormone (FSH) and luteinizing hormone (LH) from the pituitary gland?**

   a. Thyrotropin-releasing hormone (TRH)

   b. Gonadotropin-releasing hormone (GnRH)

   c. Adrenocorticotropic hormone (ACTH)

   d. Growth hormone-releasing hormone (GHRH)

79. **Which hormone does the hypothalamus release to stimulate the release of follicle-stimulating hormone (FSH) and luteinizing hormone (LH) from the pituitary gland?**

   a. Thyrotropin-releasing hormone (TRH)

   b. Gonadotropin-releasing hormone (GnRH)

   c. Adrenocorticotropic hormone (ACTH)

   d. Growth hormone-releasing hormone (GHRH)

80. **What effect does insulin have on the body?**

   a. It increases blood glucose levels

   b. It decreases blood glucose levels

   c. It increases blood pressure

   d. It decreases blood pressure

81. **Which hormone is primarily produced by alpha cells in the pancreas?**

   a. Insulin

   b. Glucagon

   c. Somatostatin

   d. Amylin

82. **What effect does glucagon have on the body?**

   a. It increases blood glucose levels

   b. It decreases blood glucose levels

   c. It increases blood pressure

   d. It decreases blood pressure

83. **Euthyroid syndrome is reported in which of the following diseases?**

   a. Rabies

   b. CD

   c. Parvo viral infection

   d. Corona viral infection

84. **What causes hypertrophy of beta cells leading to hyper-glycaemia?**

   a. Glucagon

   b. Insulin

   c. Glucocorticoids

   d. Aldosterone

85. **The alpha cells of islets of Langerhans produce:**

   a. Insulin

   b. Glucagon

   c. Somatostatin

   d. Vimentin

86. **In Hashimoto's syndrome, autoantibodies are produced against:**

   a. TSH

   b. T3

   c. T4

   d. Thyroglobulin

87. **Chronic pancreatitis in old dogs can cause :**

   a. Diabetes insipidus

   b. Diabetes mellitus

   c. Cushing's syndrome

   d. Klein filters syndrome

88. **Goitre can lead to:**

   a. Hypothyroidism

   b. Hyperthyroidism

   c. Thyroid neoplasm

   d. a and b

89. **Hyperparathyroidism is associated with:**

   a. Kidney disease

   b. Liver disease

   c. Cardiac disease

   d. Thyroid disease

90. **Seasonal oestrus in animals influences which hormone from the pineal gland?**

   a. Pituitrin

   b. Melatonin

c. Oestrogen

d. Progesterone

91. Hypocalcaemia and muscular spasm are the features of:

a. Hyperthyroidism

b. Hyperparathyroidism

c. Hypoparathyroidism

d. Hypothyroidism

92. Arteriosclerosis in animals is characterized by:

a. Hypothyroidism

b. Hyperthyroidism

c. Pancreatitis

d. a and c

93. Acromegaly is characterized by the increase in hormone from which gland?

a. Adrenal

b. Thyroid

c. Pituitary

d. Hypothalamus

94. Iodine deficiency can result in what type of goitre?

a. Nodular

b. Colloid

c. Hyperplastic

d. Familial

95. Which hormone can inhibit gastrointestinal hormones?

a. Gastrin

b. Inhibin

c. Somatostatin

d. Insulin

96. **Somatostatin is produced from which cells in the pancreas?**

   a. Alpha

   b. Beta

   c. Delta

   d. Gamma

97. **Which gland is located at the base of the cranium?**

   a. Pituitary

   b. Hypothalamus

   c. Pineal

   d. Hippocampus

98. **Increased levels of prolactin is seen in which condition?**

   a. Pituitary adenoma

   b. Pheochromocytoma

   c. Pancreatic adenoma

   d. Thyroid carcinoma

99. **Calcitonin is produced by which cells of the thyroid gland?**

   a. Beta cells

   b. C cell

   c. Alpha cells

   d. Delta ells

100. **Which of the following is a goitrogenic feed item in animals?**

   a. Cabbage

   b. Carrot

   c. Potato

   d. Tomato

Answers

1.	b	26.	b	51.	d	76.	b
2.	b	27.	d	52.	c	77.	b
3.	c	28.	a	53.	c	78.	b
4.	c	29.	c	54.	a	79.	b
5.	b	30.	c	55.	b	80.	b
6.	b	31.	a	56.	b	81.	b
7.	c	32.	a	57.	b	82.	a
8.	d	33.	c	58.	c	83.	c
9.	a	34.	b	59.	c	84.	c
10.	d	35.	a	60.	d	85.	c
11.	b	36.	b	61.	b	86.	d
12.	c	37.	c	62.	b	87.	b
13.	a	38.	a	63.	b	88.	d
14.	a	39.	a	64.	a	89.	a
15.	b	40.	a	65.	d	90.	b
16.	a	41.	b	66.	a	91.	c
17.	a	42.	c	67.	b	92.	d
18.	c	43.	b	68.	a	93.	c
19.	?d	44.	c	69.	a	94.	b
20.	c	45.	b	70	a	95.	c
21.	b	46.	a	71.	b	96.	c
22.	d	47.	d	72.	b	97.	c
23.	b	48.	d	73.	c	98.	a
24.	a	49.	b	74.	a	99.	?b
25.	a	50.	a	75.	a	100.	a

6 Diseases of the Cardiovascular System

Shashi Pradhan, Vaishali Kumre, Deepika Caeser and Madhuri Dhurvey

Introduction

The cardiovascular system comprises the heart, veins, arteries and capillary beds. The atrioventricular (mitral and tricuspid) and semilunar (aortic and pulmonic) valves keep blood flowing in one direction through the heart, and valves in large veins keep blood flowing back toward the heart. The rate and force of contraction of the heart and the degree of constriction or dilatation of blood vessels are determined by the autonomic nervous system (sympathetic and parasympathetic) and hormones produced either by the heart and blood vessels (i.e. paracrine or autocrine) or at a distance from the heart and blood vessels (i.e. endocrine).

Cardiac diseases can be either congenital defects or acquired in nature. The diseases of greatest importance, because of their prevalence, are mitral regurgitation in dogs (degenerative mitral valve disease), hypertrophic cardiomyopathy in cats, dilated cardiomyopathy (DCM) in dogs, arrhythmogenic right ventricular cardiomyopathy in boxers and bulldogs, and heartworm disease.

Auscultation of a cardiac murmur can indicate underlying structural cardiac disease or a physiologic change (e.g. elevated cardiac output). A heart murmur is generated by turbulent blood flow that can be auscultated with a stethoscope.

Any cardiac rhythm falling outside the normal sinus rhythm is termed an arrhythmia. Arrhythmias develop secondary to underlying structural heart disease, abnormalities of electrical pathways or secondary to extracardiac causes. An arrhythmia that is too fast, too slow, or too irregular can result in reduced cardiac output, thereby causing clinical signs that could include exercise intolerance, syncope or exacerbation of congestive heart failure (CHF).

© CAB International 2024. *Key Questions in Clinical Farm Animal Medicine Volume 1: Principles of Disease Examination, Diagnosis and Management* (ed. T. Rana)
DOI: 10.1079/9781800624788.0006

Heart failure (HF) is the terminal event of heart disease. Progressive, adaptive changes in the neurohormonal axis develop and have multiple negative effects on the myocardium and cardiac output. Clinical signs of HF in cattle are a consequence of increased hydrostatic pressure and peripheral oedema. The prognosis of heart disease (HD) is poor when clinical signs of HF are observed. The prognosis of HD in cattle is classically reported to be guarded to poor even if HF is absent.

Multiple Choice Questions

1. **A slow heart rate is known as**

    a. Bradycardia

    b. Tachycardia

    c. Hypocardia

    d. Hypercardia

2. **Gallop rhythm is observed in:**

    a. Horses

    b. Cattle

    c. Both

    d. None of these

3. **Pulsation of the jugular vein is observed at:**

    a. 5–8 cm above the level of the apex of the heart

    b. The mitral valve

    c. 5–8 cm above the level of the base of the head

    d. The tricuspid valve

4. **Absence and presence (A wave) atrial contraction is observed in:**

    a. Primary heart block

    b. Secondary heart block

    c. a and b

    d. None of these

5. **Which signs are indicative of cardiac insufficiency?**

    a. Dyspnoea

    b. Fatigue

    c. Prolonged elevation in heart rate

    d. All of these

6. **Electrocardiography represents:**
   a. Depolarization
   b. Electrical activity of the heart
   c. Repolarization
   d. None of these

7. **The concentration of cardiac troponin I in healthy neonatal foals is:**
   a. < 0.49 ng/ml
   b. < 0.15 ng/ml
   c. 0.75 ng/ml
   d. < 0.84 ng/ml

8. **Healthy cattle have a cardiac troponin I concentration of:**
   a. < 0.49 ng/ml
   b. < 0.04 ng/ml
   c. 0.64 ng/ml
   d. < 0.78 ng/ml

9. **Stroke volume is:**
   a. SV= cardiac output × heart rate
   b. SV = cardiac output + heart rate
   c. SV = cardiac output / heart rate
   d. SV= cardiac output - heart rate

10. **Cardiac output can be measured by:**
    a. Thermodilution technique
    b. Doppler echocardiography
    c. a and b
    d. None of these

11. **Right-sided heart failure causes:**
    a. Interstitial oedema in the lungs
    b. Increase in jugular venous pressure

    c. Increase in pulmonary venous pressure

    d. None of these

12. **The atrioventricular valves close preventing backflow of blood into:**

    a. The atria during diastole and filling

    b. The atria during systole and emptying

    c. The ventricles during diastole and filling

    d. The ventricles during systole and emptying

13. **Which type of blood cell is involved in the clotting mechanism of blood?**

    a. Neutrophils

    b. Eosinophils

    c. Lymphocytes

    d. Platelets

14. **Cardiovascular dysfunction can be due to:**

    a. Cardiac arrythmia

    b. Obstructed blood flow

    c. Regurgitant flow

    d. All of the above

15. **Left-sided heart failure causes an:**

    a. Increase in pulmonary venous pressure

    b. Decrease in pulmonary venous pressure

    c. Increase in pulmonary arterial pressure

    d. Decrease in pulmonary arterial pressure

16. **Sudden cessation of heartbeat leads to which of the following?**

    i. Acute heart failure

    ii. Decrease in cardiac output

    iii. Congestive heart failure

a. i, ii, iii

b. ii, iii

c. i, iii

d. i, ii

17. **Circuit failure can be due to:**

a. Hypovolemic shock

b. Pooling of blood in peripheral vessels

c. Increased capillary permeability

d. All of these

18. **The effects of circuit failure are the same as:**

a. Acute heart failure

b. Congestive heart failure

c. Neither a nor b

d. a and b

19. **The tendency of the heart to increase its output several fold in response to normal physiological demands is called:**

a. Cardiac output

b. Stroke volume

c. Cardiac reserve

d. None of these

20. **Cardiac output is the:**

a. Sum of heart rate and stroke volume

b. Product of heart and stroke volume

c. Sum of heart rate and cardiac reserve

d. Product of heart rate and cardiac reserve

21. **The maximum heart rate in trained horses is how many times the resting value?**

a. 6–7

b. 1–2

c. 14–15

d. 2–4

22. **Approximately what percentage of carbon dioxide is found in expired air?**

a. 0.04%

b. 20%

c. 5%

d. 40%

23. **The maximum heart rate in cattle is how many times the resting value?**

a. 6–7

b. 2–4

c. 14–15

d. 1–2

24. **Angiotensin II is:**

a. A vasodilator that promotes the effect of norepinephrine

b. A vasoconstrictor that promotes the effect of norepinephrine

c. A vasoconstrictor that inhibits the effect of norepinephrine

d. A vasodilator that inhibits the effect of norepinephrine

25. **What is the 'crux' of veterinary medicine?**

a. Anamnesis

b. Diagnosis

c. Inspection

d. Prognosis

26. **An increase in the amplitude of the pulse can be due to:**

a. Increase in cardiac stroke volume

b. Decrease in cardiac stroke volume

c. Reduced venous return

d. Reduced contractile power of the heart

27. **The ratio of heart weight to body weight is:**
    a. Greater in athletic animals than in unathletic animals
    b. Less in athletic animals than unathletic animals
    c. The same in both
    d. The same irrespective of athletic activity

28. **Cardiac hypertrophy is the usual response to:**
    a. Decreased pressure load
    b. Increased pressure load
    c. Decreased volume load
    d. Increased volume load

29. **Eccentric hypertrophy is the usual response to:**
    a. Increased volume load
    b. Decreased volume load
    c. Increased pressure load
    d. Decreased pressure load

30. **Which of the following clinical signs is most likely to be present in a cat with heart disease?**
    a. Anorexia
    b. Coughing
    c. Excessive urination
    d. Subcutaneous oedema

31. **What is the right ventricle more capable of sustaining than the left ventricle?**
    a. Flow load
    b. Volume load
    c. Pressure load
    d. All of these

32. **What is the left ventricle more capable of sustaining than the right ventricle?**

   a. Pressure load

   b. Volume load

   c. Flow load

   d. All of these

33. **Arrhythmias are the common cause of:**

   a. CHF

   b. AHF

   c. a and b

   d. None of these

34. **Venous congestion in the portal system is a sequel of:**

   a. Hepatic congestion

   b. Hepatic dilation

   c. Renal congestion

   d. Renal dilation

35. **Due to G suit, ruminants do not suffer oedema in the legs as a result of:**

   a. Right-sided heart failure

   b. Left-sided heart failure

   c. a and b

   d. None of these

36. **Which of these administration methods are suitable for digoxin?**

   i. IV

   ii. IM

   iii. Orally

   a. i, iii

   b. i, ii

c. i, ii, iii

d. None of these

37. **The half-life of digoxin in cattle is:**

    a. 2–3 hours

    b. 5.5–7.2 hours

    c. 30 minutes

    d. 48 hours

38. **Heart sounds are associated with valve closure. They occur because of the rapid changes in the speed of blood flow and vibrations throughout the heart, valves, and the cardia blood. There are four heart sounds that can potentially be auscultated, but they are not normally heard in all species. All four heart sounds are most likely to be heard in healthy animals of which of the following species?**

    a. Cats

    b. Dogs

    c. Ferrets

    d. Horses

39. **Myxomatous degeneration of the mitral valve is the most common cardiac disease of dogs. Dogs with early and middle stage of disease do not typically show clinical signs other than a systolic murmur. When regurgitation develops and becomes severe, heart failure ensues. Which of the following clinical signs is least likely in a dog with heart failure caused by mitral valve degeneration?**

    a. Ascites

    b. Exercise intolerance

    c. Syncope

    d. Tachypnoea

40. **The drug of choice for endocarditis is:**

    a. Sulphur

    b. Chloramphenicol

c. Tetracycline

d. Penicillin

41. **Slowest conduction velocity occurs in**

a. Atrium

b. AV node

c. Bundle of Hiss

d. Purkinjee fibre

42. **The purpose of having valves in the cardiovascular system is to:**

a. Provide sound so that the heart health can be monitored

b. Ensure blood flows in one direction

c. Prevent blood from flowing too quickly

d. Regulate blood pressure

43. **Muffling of the heart sound is due to an increase between the heart and the stethoscope in:**

a. Tissue

b. Tissue and tissue interfaces

c. Tissue and muscles

d. Muscles

44. **Accentuated C wave occurs with:**

a. Bicuspid valve insufficiency

b. Bicuspid valve stenosis

c. Tricuspid valve insufficiency

d. Tricuspid valve stenosis

45. **The recording speed of an ECG is:**

a. 25 mm/sec

b. 50 mm/sec

c. 75 mm/sec

d. 100 mm/sec

46. **Foetal electrocardiography can determine:**

    a. Whether a foetus is live or dead

    b. The presence of a singleton or twins

    c. Foetal distress during prolonged parturition

    d. All of these

47. **The foetal heart rate for calves during advancing pregnancy:**

    a. Does not decrease

    b. Does not increase

    c. Decreases

    d. Increases

48. **A decrease in amplitude and flattening of the P wave, widening of the QRS complex and an increased symmetry and amplitude of the T wave are seen in:**

    a. Hypocalcaemia

    b. Hypercalcemia

    c. Hypokalaemia

    d. Hyperkalaemia

49. **The serum concentration of what provides an excellent cardiac biomarker in large animals?**

    a. Cardiac troponin I

    b. Cardiac troponin C

    c. Cardiac troponin T

    d. None of these

50. **Of the following statements:**

    i. Cardiac troponin C has greater myocardial selectivity than Cardiac troponin T

    ii. Cardiac troponin T is a preferred biomarker

    a. Statement i is correct Statement ii is incorrect

    b. Statement ii is correct Statement i is incorrect

    c. Both statements are correct

    d. Both statements are incorrect

51. **The half-life of digoxin in horses is:**

    a. 2–3 hours

    b. 17–23 hours

    c. 30 minutes

    d. 48 hours

52. **Previously healthy puppies begin vomiting when first fed on solid food. There is no fever and when immediately returned to a liquid diet, no vomiting occurs. The congenital anomaly of the cardiovascular system involved here is:**

    a. Persistence of right aortic arch

    b. Subaortic septal defect

    c. Dextro rotation of aorta

    d. Patent foramen ovale

53. **Vegetative endocarditis may be one of the lesions found in:**

    a. Bovine traumatic gastritis

    b. Equine viral arteritis

    c. Swine erysipelas

    d. Hog cholera

54. **Trimethoprim-sulphonamides combinations are usually available in the ratio of:**

    a. 1:1

    b. 1:5

    c. 1:3

    d. 1:7

55. **The normal pH of bovine blood ranges between:**

    a. 6.6–6.8

    b. 6.9–7.1

c. 7.2–7.4

d. 7.5–77

56. Digoxin is most commonly used in the treatment of:

a. Pericarditis

b. Endocarditis

c. Congestive heart failure

d. None of these

57. Shock occurs after:

a. Trauma

b. CHF

c. Heart failure

d. Oedema

58. Shock is manifested by:

a. Death

b. Circulatory failure

c. Peripheral circulatory failure

d. None of these

59. Which aspect of clinical examination is the most important?

a. Animal

b. History

c. Environment

d. None of these

60. The jugular pulse is an important feature in:

a. Milk fever

b. Acute heart failure

c. CHF

d. Traumatic reticulo peritonitis

61. **Traumatic pericarditis is associated with which of the following?**

   a. Pronounced leucocytosis

   b. Pronounced leucocytosis with neutrophilia

   c. Pronounced leucocytosis with neutropenia

   d. None of these

62. **In shock we see:**

   a. Peripheral circulatory failure

   b. Increase in blood pressure

   c. Increase in total blood volume

   d. All of these

63. **Anaemia is clinically characterized by:**

   a. Tachycardia

   b. Muscle weakness

   c. Pale mucus membranes

   d. All of these

64. **Which sulphonamides are mostly used in large animals**

   a. Sulfadiazine

   b. Sulfaguanidine

   c. Sulfamezathine

   d. None of these

65. **A blood picture characterized by the presence of reticulocytes, polychromatic macrocytes and nucleated erythrocytes indicates:**

   a. Aplastic anaemia

   b. Abnormal erythropoiesis

   c. Normal erythropoiesis

   d. Mylopthisicanaemia

66. **In farm animals, the only common form of leukaemia is:**

    a. Hyelogenous leukaemia

    b. Haemopoietic tissue tumours

    c. Lymphomatosis

    d. Myelopthisic anaemia

67. **In cases of high leucocyte count, the disease may be:**

    a. Localized generalized bacterial infection

    b. Leukaemia

    c. Lymphomatosis

    d. Bone marrow depression

68. **Spontaneous haemorrhages of fatal origin in domestic animals may arise from:**

    a. Traumatic pericarditis

    b. Acute heamonchus infection

    c. Warfarin and sweat clover poisoning

    d. Rupture of the middle uterine artery during prolapse of uterus

69. **Besides reduced hematocrit and reduced haemoglobin concentration in blood, an additional indication confirming fatal haemorrhage is:**

    a. Reduced total erythrocytic count

    b. Reduced platelet count

    c. Increased bleeding time

    d. Increased clotting and prothrombin time

70. **Bovine blood can be stored at 6 °C for safe transfusion without losing much beneficial effect for up to:**

    a. 1 month

    b. 10 days

    c. 1 week

    d. 2 weeks

71. **A 'tiger heart' appearance in the cardiac muscles occurs in which disease?**

   a. Foot and mouth disease

   b. Rinderpest

   c. a and b

   d. Ephemeral fever

72. **Vascular endocarditis occurs in which disease?**

   a. Ephemeral fever

   b. Bluetongue

   c. Swine fever

   d. All of these

73. **Heartwater disease is caused by:**

   a. *Cowdria ruminatium*

   b. Equine influenza

   c. *Moraxella bovis*

   d. All of these

74. **The level of calcium in normal blood is:**

   a. 1–2 mg %

   b. 2–6 mg %

   c. 6–8 mg %

   d. 9–10 mg %

75. **Normal ratio of calcium to phosphorus in blood is:**

   a. 2:1

   b. 4:1

   c. 6:1

   d. 8:1

76. **The normal ratio of calcium to magnesium in blood is:**

   a. 2:1

   b. 4:1

c. 6:1

d. 8:1

77. **Increased heart rate with detectable influence is known as:**

   a. Simple tachycardia

   b. Paroxysmal tachycardia

   c. a and b

   d. None of these

78. **What is the normal level of P in blood?**

   a. 0.5–3 mg/100 ml

   b. 3–5 mg/100 ml

   c. 4–7 mg/100ml

   d. 5–9 mg/100ml

79. **An increase heart rate without detectable influence is known as:**

   a. Simple tachycardia

   b. Paroxysmal tachycardia

   c. a and b

   d. None of these

80. **Which tachycardia is common in horses:**

   a. Simple tachycardia

   b. Paroxysmal tachycardia

   c. a and b

   d. None of these

81. **DOC of arrhythmia in large animals is:**

   a. Lidocaine

   b. Bromocaine

   c. a and b

   d. None of these

82. **In an electrocardiogram, ventricular tachycardia shows:**

    a. Inverted P wave

    b. Prolonged ST interval

    c. Multiple QRS complex

    d. None of these

83. **The drug of choice for horses with ventricular tachycardia is quinidine:**

    a. Sulphate

    b. Nitrate

    c. a and b

    d. None of these

84. **A good alternative for quinidine sulphate in horses is:**

    a. Phenyrin sodium

    b. Quinidine chloride

    c. a and b

    d. None of these

85. **Antiarrhythmic agents act by blocking what?**

    a. Potassium channels

    b. Sodium channels

    c. a and b

    d. None of these

86. **The half-life of lignocaine is:**

    a. 1 minute

    b. 30 minutes

    c. 20 minutes

    d. 40 minutes

87. **What is the effect of exercise on the circulatory system?**

    a. Increased stroke volume

    b. Increase in heart size

    c. Decreased cholesterol level

    d. All of these

88. **What is determined by ECG?**

    a. Mechanical performance of the heart

    b. Systolic and diastolic information

    c. Cardiac output

    d. Effects due to changes in fluid electrolytes

89. **How long does it take for phenodyroin to exert an anti-arrhythmic effect?**

    a. 2–6 hours

    b. 17–20 hours

    c. 48 hours

    d. 72 hours

90. **A P wave may be detected in an electrocardiogram but has what relationship with QRS complex?**

    a. Linear

    b. Hyperbolic

    c. Parabolic

    d. No relation

91. **All of the following are types of leucocytes, except:**

    a. Lymphocytes

    b. Monocytes

    c. Eosinophils

    d. Erythrocytes

92. **Which of the following pairs has a double circulation pathway?**

   a. Amphibians and mammals

   b. Reptiles and mammals

   c. Birds and mammals

   d. Fishes and birds

93. **Which blood group has no antibody?**

   a. O

   b. A

   c. AB

   d. B

94. **Which part of the body can be called a kind of 'blood bank'?**

   a. Heart

   b. Liver

   c. Spleen

   d. Lungs

95. **Which of the following has a closed type of circulatory system?**

   a. Cockroaches

   b. Fish

   c. Mollusca

   d. Scorpions

96. **The most potent vasoconstrictor is:**

   a. Endothelin

   b. Vasopressin

   c. Substrate P

   d. Platelet activating factor

97. **If uncountered, ventricular tachycardia may lead to:**

   a. Ventricular fibrillation

   b. Death

   c. a and b

   d. None of these

98. A major disadvantage of lignocaine is its:

   a. Short duration of action

   b. High availability

   c. Long duration of action

   d. All of these

99. Movement of leucocytes from blood capillaries is known as

   a. Amoeboid movement

   b. Chemotaxis

   c. Diapedesis

   d. Brownian movement

100. The duration of action of lignocaine is less than that of:

   a. Phenodyoin

   b. Bromocaine

   c. a and b

   d. None of these

101. Who developed the electrocardiogram?

   a. Wilhelm His

   b. Hubert Mann

   c. Niels Bohr

   d. Willem Einthoven

102. What does a P wave represent?

   a. Depolarization of the atria

   b. Repolarization of the ventricles

   c. Depolarization of the ventricles

   d. Depolarization of the atria

103. **Antiarrhythmic agents shorten the respiratory period of the:**

    a. Myocardial tissues

    b. Endocardial tissues

    c. a and b

    d. None of these

104. **Lidocaine has what level of cardiovascular toxicity?**

    a. High

    b. Moderate

    c. Low

    d. None of these

105. **Which of these can be used for the treatment of ventricular arrythmia?**

    a. Magnesium sulphate

    b. Sodium chloride

    c. a and b

    d. None of these

106. **Muscular fasciculation is the initial sign of what type of toxicity?**

    a. Quinodine nitrate

    b. Quinodine sulphate

    c. Quinodine chloride

    d. None of these

107. **Vegetative endocarditis may be one of the chief lesions appearing in:**

    a. Bovine traumatic gastritis

    b. Swine erysipelas

    c. Equine viral arthritis

    d. Hog cholera

108. **Digoxin is most commonly used in the treatment of:**

    a. Pericarditis

    b. Endocarditis

    c. CHF

    d. None of these

109. **The most accurate definition of artery is:**

    a. A vessel that carries highly oxygenated blood

    b. A vessel that contains smooth muscles

    c. A vessel that transports blood away from the heart

    d. A vessel that transports blood towards the heart

110. **Traumatic pericarditis is associated with which of the following?**

    a. Pronounced leucocytosis

    b. Pronounced leucocytosis with neutrophilia

    c. Pronounced leucocytosis with neutropenia

    d. None of these

111. **Haemophilia B occurs due to the deficiency of**

    a. Coagulation factor VII

    b. Coagulation factor IX

    c. Coagulation factor VIII

    d. Coagulation factor X

112. **Pulmonary oedema in animals is seen as equating with:**

    a. CHF

    b. ANTU poisoning

    c. Acute anaphylaxis

    d. All of these

113. **Diagnosis of bovine lymphosarcoma should depend upon:**

    a. Haemogram

    b. Abnormal lymphocytes

    c. a and b

    d. Haemogram, bone marrow and histopathological changes

114. **Which of the following is a true oxidation product of haemoglobin?**

    a. Oxyhaemoglobin

    b. Methaemoglobin

    c. Carboxy haemoglobulin

    d. Carbaminohaemoglobin

115. **The presence of leptocytes in blood film suggests:**

    a. Aplastic anaemia

    b. Haemorrhagic anaemia

    c. Granulocytic leukaemia

    d. Pernicious anaemia

116. **Osmoreceptors are present in**

    a. Hypothalamus

    b. Medulla

    c. Heart

    d. Kidney

117. **Bone marrow diagnosis is a method is for the confirmation of leukaemia in:**

    a. Buffalo

    b. Horses

    c. Sheep and goats

    d. Cows

118. **The earliest signs of the development of leukaemia in dairy animals is development of lesions in:**

    a. The lymph nodes

    b. The spleen

    c. Peripheral blood

    d. Bone marrow

119. **Leukaemia in domestic animals can be described as:**

    a. A metabolic arrangement

    b. A bovine leukosis viral infection

    c. Neoplastic in origin

    d. Immunogenic incompatibility

120. **In trypanosomiasis and anaplasmosis, the cause of anaemia is:**

    a. Haemolytic

    b. Haemorrhagic

    c. Caused by an increase in phagocytosis by the spleen

    d. An Ag-Ab complex reaction leading to haemolysis intravenously

121. **In healthy animals, the rate of intake of iron from digested gastrointestinal tract content into the circulation is:**

    a. 8%

    b. 10%

    c. Less than 1%

    d. 15%

122. **The oral daily dose of iron preparation in anaemic cattle is:**

    a. 20–25 g

    b. 5–10 g

    c. 25–30 g

    d. 50–60 g

123. **What is observable in co-deficiency?**

    a. Microcytic hypochromic anaemia

    b. Normocytic normochromic anaemia

    c. Macrocytic hypochromic anaemia

    d. Macrocytic normochromic anaemia

124. **Besides hypovolemia and anaemic anoxia, the pathogenesis of acute haemorrhage includes:**

    a. Peripheral circulatory failure

    b. Loss of plasma protein

    c. Decrease in blood supply from splenic stores

    d. Decrease in osmotic pressure of running blood

125. **In piglets with iron deficiency anaemia, typical alarming symptoms after transfusion of incompatible blood include:**

    a. Salivation

    b. Muscular tremors

    c. Hiccup and coughing

    d. High rise of temperature

126. **Cytokines are:**

    a. Low molecular weight proteins

    b. Enzymes

    c. Autocoids

    d. Immunoglobins

127. **An erythrocytic compatibility test is the best indicator of survival of donor blood in:**

    a. Swine

    b. Bovines

    c. Canines

    d. Equines

128. **Heinz body formation associated with haemolytic anaemia is reported in horses poisoned by:**

    a. Selenium

    b. Lead

    c. Phenothiazine

    d. Mercury

129. **Heinz body haemolytic anaemia may occur due to a deficiency of:**

    a. Alkaline phosphatase

    b. Cholinestease

    c. Glucose-6 Phosphate dehydrogenase

    d. 6-G-H glucosides

130. **After splenomegaly, the quine erythrocytes may contain what percentage of Heinz bodies?**

    a. 1%

    b. 15%

    c. 10%

    d. 25%

131. **Congenital porphyria of cattle is caused by:**

    a. Defective haemoglobin synthesis

    b. Accumulation of uroporphyrins

    c. Hepatotoxicosis

    d. Accumulation of coproporphyrins

132. **In bracken fern poisoning, a typical blood picture includes:**

    a. Anaemic erythrocytes

    b. Reticulocytes

    c. Leucocytosis

    d. Neutrophilia

133. **In autoimmune haemolytic anaemia, what effect do macro-phages have?**

    a. Increase pathogenesis of erythrocytes

    b. Phagocytosis of erythrocytes devoid of opsonic antibodies

    c. Sequestration of monocytes

    d. Splenic hypersensitivity

134. **Which form of swine erysipelas disease is characterized by suppurative and vegetative endocarditis?**

    a. Acute

    b. Chronic

    c. a and b

    d. None of these

135. **Left-sided heart failure is characterized by:**

    a. Dyspnoea

    b. Alteration of pulse

    c. Coughing

    d. All of these

136. **Which is a drug of choice in cardiac disorders?**

    a. Verapmil

    b. Captopril

    c. Prazosin

    d. All of these

137. **What is a differential diagnosis of foreign body syndrome?**

    a. Tetanus

    b. Abomasal impaction

    c. Vagal Indigestion

    d. All of these

138. **An animal presented with reduced ruminal movement, muf-fled heart sound, snuffling noise in the heart, brisket oedema and jugular pulse is likely to be suffering from:**

    a. TRP

    b. Endocarditis

    c. Myocarditis

    d. Pericarditis

139. **Which is a common cardiac disease associated with murmur?**

    a. Functional murmur

    b. Pulmonic stenosis

    c. Patent ductus arteriosus

    d. All of these

140. **Dose endocarditis affects the:**

    a. Lining of the heart

    b. Lining of the heart and heart valves

    c. Lining of the heart valves

    d. None of these

141. **The clinical pathology of myocarditis shows:**

    a. Increased SGOT, decreased SGPT, increased lactic dehydrogenase

    b. Increased SGOT, increased SGPT, increased lactic dehydrogenase

    c. Decreased SGOT, increased SGPT, decreased lactic dehydrogenase

    d. Decreased SGOT, decreased SGP, increased lactic dehydrogenase

142. **Which type of respiration is seen in CHF?**

    a. Chyne stroke

    b. Biots type

    c. a and b

    d. None of these

143. **Gallop rhythm over the mitral valve is seen in:**

    a. Right-side heart failure

    b. Endocarditis

    c. Left-side heart failure

    d. Pericarditis

144. **An increased arterial rate (200–400 beats per minute), with an increased ventricular rate (100–200 beats per minute) is known as:**

    a. Gallop rhythm

    b. Atrial flutter

    c. Ventricular fibrillation

    d. Sinus arrythmia

145. **Uncoordinated twitching of the ventricle is known as:**

    a. Gallop rhythm

    b. Atrial flutter

    c. Ventricular fibrillation

    d. Sinus arrythmia

146. **Which condition occurs as a result of sudden calcium infusion?**

    a. Gallop rhythm

    b. Atrial flutter

    c. Ventricular fibrillation

    d. Sinus arrythmia

147. **What is radiotelemetry?**

    a. Use of an ECG machine

    b. Effect of radioactivity on the heart

    c. Study of radio isotopes

    d. None of these

148. **Which dye is used to test circulatory output?**

    a. Trypan blue (T-1354)

    b. Evan blue (T-1824)

    c. Methylene blue

    d. All of these

149. **By X-ray examination we can detect:**

    a. Enlargement of the heart

    b. Displacement of the heart

    c. Hydropericardium

    d. All of these

150. **A BP instrument is known as a:**

    a. Baumanometer

    b. Sphygmomanometer

    c. a and b

    d. None of these

151. **Vasovagal syncope occurs due to:**

    a. Reduced stimulation of the vagus nerve

    b. Overstimulation of the vagus nerve

    c. Failure of transmission of the wave impulse through the heart

    d. Contraction of the atrium at a very rapid rate

152. **Atrial fibrillation is due to:**

    a. Reduced stimulation of the vagus nerve

    b. Overstimulation of the vagus nerve

    c. Failure of transmission of the wave impulse through the heart

    d. Contraction of atrium at a very rapid rate

153. **Heart block is due to:**

    a. Reduced stimulation of the vagus nerve

    b. Overstimulation of the vagus nerve

    c. Failure of transmission of the wave impulse through the heart

    d. Contraction of the atrium at a very rapid rate

154. **Pain of percussion of cardiac area (3–5 intercoastal space) and increased cardiac dullness is characteristic of:**

    a. Pericarditis

    b. Myocarditis

    c. a and b

    d. None of these

155. **Stenosis of the tricuspid valve leads to:**

    a. Positive jugular pulse

    b. Negative jugular pulse

    c. a and b

    d. None of these

156. **Insufficiency of the tricuspid valve leads to:**

    a. Positive jugular pulse

    b. Negative jugular pulse

    c. a and b

    d. None of these

157. **Which condition occurs in pericarditis, traumatic pericarditis and chronic heart failure?**

    a. Positive jugular pulse

    b. Negative jugular pulse

    c. a and b

    d. None of these

158. **The cause of death in traumatic pericarditis is:**

    a. Asphyxia

    b. Toxaemia

    c. a and b

    d. None of these

159.   **The exercise tolerance in traumatic pericarditis is:**

   a. Excellent

   b. Poor

   c. Good

   d. None of these

160.   **Which condition occurs in advanced pregnancy and after parturition?**

   a. Traumatic pericarditis

   b. Myocarditis

   c. Endometritis

   d. All of these

161.   **Arrhythmicity of the heart is known as:**

   a. Gallop rhythm

   b. Ventricular fibrillation

   c. Atrial flutter

   d. Sinus arrythmia

162.   **Reduplication of 1 and 3 heart rate is known as:**

   a. Gallop rhythm

   b. Ventricular fibrillation

   c. Atrial flutter

   d. Sinus arrythmia

163.   **In which condition does oedema of the conjunctiva result in grape-like masses hanging from the eyelid?**

   a. Traumatic pericarditis

   b. Myocarditis

   c. Endometritis

   d. All of these

164. **The sound of pericarditis is:**
    a. First frictional
    b. Tinkling
    c. Second splashing or gurgling
    d. All of these

165. **Generalized oedema occurs in:**
    a. Pericarditis
    b. Endocarditis, myocarditis
    c. Pericarditis, endocarditis, myocarditis
    d. None of these

166. **Oedema of the brisket region is a characteristic symptom of:**
    a. Pericarditis
    b. Pericarditis, endocarditis, myocarditis
    c. Endocarditis, myocarditis
    d. None of these

167. **Cardiac murmur occurs in:**
    a. Pericarditis
    b. Endocarditis, myocarditis
    c. Pericarditis, endocarditis, myocarditis
    d. None of these

168. **Cardiac murmur is found in which disease?**
    a. Endocarditis, diaphragmatic hernia
    b. Choke
    c. Tympany
    d. All of these

169. **Band cells are immature:**
    a. Eosinophils
    b. Basophils

   c. Neutrophils

   d. Monocytes

170. **The dose of penicillin for treatment of endocarditis is:**

   a. 1000 IU/kg BWT

   b. 10,000 IU/kg BWT

   c. 5000 IU/kg BWT

   d. 20,000 IU/kg BWT

171. **Sudden filling of the pericardial sac is known as:**

   a. Cardiac tamponade

   b. Cardiac syncope

   c. a and b

   d. None of these

172. **A transient attack of acute heart failure is manifested as:**

   a. Cardiac tamponade

   b. Cardiac syncope

   c. a and b

   d. None of these

173. **HLA antigens are found in**

   a. All leucocytes

   b. B cells

   c. T cells

   d. All nucleated cells

174. **'Tiger heart' is a post-mortem lesion of which disease?**

   a. Pericarditis

   b. Endocarditis

   c. Myocarditis

   d. Peripheral circulatory failure

175. **In which disease is there is no post-mortem lesion?**

   a. Pericarditis

   b. Myocarditis

   c. Endocarditis

   d. Peripheral circulatory failure

176. **Cauliflower-like growth or vegetative growth is a post-mortem lesion of which disease?**

   a. Pericarditis

   b. Endocarditis

   c. Myocarditis

   d. Peripheral circulatory failure

177. **Oedema, positive jugular pulse, palpable enlarged liver and concentrated urine are symptoms of:**

   a. Right-side CHF

   b. Left-side CHF

   c. a & b

   d. None of these

178. **Presence of murmur and moist rales at the base of the lungs are symptoms of:**

   a. Right-side CHF

   b. Left-side CHF

   c. a and b

   d. None of these

179. **Which is absent in CHF but present in TP?**

   a. Metallic sound

   b. Leucocytosis

   c. Neutrophilia, shift to left

   d. All of these

180. **Digitalization is performed in which animal?**

    a. Dogs

    b. Horses

    c. Ruminants

    d. All of these

181. **Failure of the venous return system, resulting in pooling of blood in the vein with vasodilation, is known as:**

    a. Acute heart failure

    b. Peripheral circulatory failure

    c. Cardiac syncope

    d. All of these

182. **In peripheral circulatory failure, if total volume is normal then it is known as:**

    a. Vasogenic peripheral circulatory failure

    b. Haemogenic peripheral circulatory failure

    c. a and b

    d. None of these

183. **In peripheral circulatory failure, if total volume is reduced then it is known as:**

    a. Vasogenic peripheral circulatory failure

    b. Haemogenic peripheral circulatory failure

    c. a and b

    d. None of these

184. **Inflammation of the lymph vessel is known as:**

    a. Lymphadenitis

    b. Lymphangitis

    c. Lymphoma

    d. All of these

185. **The hepatic portal vein carries blood away from the:**

    a. Digestive tract

    b. Liver

    c. Kidney

    d. Heart

186. **Which of the following is pulmonary hypertension?**

    a. Hypertension below sea level

    b. Hypertension at high altitude

    c. a and b

    d. None of these

187. **In which disease is the lymphatic system involved?**

    a. Leukaemia

    b. Leukopenia

    c. Leucoma

    d. Leucocytosis

188. **Which is a valvular disease?**

    a. Endocarditis

    b. Rupture of valve and valve chordae

    c. CHF

    d. All of these

189. **What is the effect of congestive heart failure on the lungs?**

    a. Pulmonary venous congestion

    b. Exercise intolerance

    c. Increased respiration rate

    d. All of these

190. **Rouleaux formation is accelerated by**

    a. Globulin

    b. Fibrinogen

c. a and b

d. Albumin

191.   In horses, epistaxis may indicate what?

a. Peripheral cardiac failure

b. Anaemia

c. Congestive heart failure

d. Lymphangitis

192.   Which is a characteristic symptom of congestive heart failure?

a. Gallop rhythm of mitral valve

b. Systolic murmur

c. Apical impulse

d. All of these

193.   The urine of congestive heart failure patients is high in:

a. Ketone

b. Glucose

c. Albumin

d. All of these

194.   What is given as treatment for congestive heart failure?

a. Diuretics

b. Vein section

c. Digitalization

d. All of these

195.   How much blood is drawn in vein section?

a. 2–4 ml lb/Body weight

b. 20–40ml lb/Body weight

c. 10–20 ml lb/Body weight

d. 100–120 ml lb/Body weight

196. **Anaemia is caused by:**

   a. Decreased concentration of RBC

   b. Decreased haemoglobin

   c. a and b

   d. None of these

197. **Which type of anaemia occurs in babesiosis, anaplasmosis and bacillary haemoglobinuria?**

   a. Microcytic hypochromic

   b. Macrocytic hypochromic

   c. Macrocytic normochromic

   d. Microcytic normochromic

198. **Systolic murmurs, which are present in anaemia, are also known as:**

   a. Haemic murmurs

   b. Anaemic murmurs

   c. a and b

   d. None of these

199. **Which type of anaemia occurs in sweet clover poisoning?**

   a. Macrocytic hypochromic

   b. Normocytic hypochromic

   c. Normocytic normochromic

   d. Microcytic hypochromic

200. **CHF is the cause of which type of renal failure?**

   a. Pre-renal

   b. Post-renal

   c. Renal

   d. All of these

Answers

1.	a	31.	a	61.	b	91.	d
2.	c	32.	a	62.	a	92.	c
3.	c	33.	b	63.	d	93.	c
4.	c	34.	a	64.	a	94.	c
5.	d	35.	a	65.	b	95.	b
6.	b	36.	a	66.	b	96.	a
7.	a	37.	b	67.	a	97.	c
8.	b	38.	d	68.	d	98.	a
9.	c	39.	a	69.	d	99.	c
10.	c	40.	d	70.	c	100.	c
11.	b	41.	b	71.	a	101.	d
12.	d	42.	b	72.	b	102.	a
13.	d	43.	b	73.	a	103.	a
14.	d	44.	c	74.	d	104.	a
15.	a	45.	a	75.	a	105.	a
16.	c	46.	d	76.	b	106.	b
17.	d	47.	b	77.	a	107.	b
18.	b	48.	d	78.	c	108.	c
19.	c	49.	a	79.	b	109.	c
20.	b	50.	d	80.	b	110.	b
21.	c	51.	c	81.	a	111.	b
22.	c	52.	a	82.	c	112.	d
23.	b	53.	b	83.	a	113.	d
24.	b	54.	c	84.	a	114.	b
25.	b	55.	c	85.	a	115.	a
26.	a	56.	c	86.	a	116.	a
27.	a	57.	a	87.	a	117.	d
28.	b	58.	c	88.	d	118.	d
29.	a	59.	b	89.	a	119.	c
30.	a	60.	d	90.	a	120.	d

(Continued)

121.	c	**141.**	d	**161.**	d	**181.**	b
122.	d	**142.**	d	**162.**	a	**182.**	a
123.	b	**143.**	d	**163.**	a	**183.**	b
124.	a	**144.**	b	**164.**	d	**184.**	b
125.	c	**145.**	c	**165.**	c	**185.**	a
126.	a	**146.**	c	**166.**	a	**186.**	b
127.	d	**147.**	a	**167.**	b	**187.**	a
128.	c	**148.**	b	**168.**	d	**188.**	d
129.	d	**149.**	d	**169.**	c	**189.**	d
130.	a	**150.**	c	**170.**	d	**190.**	c
131.	a	**151.**	b	**171.**	a	**191.**	c
132.	b	**152.**	d	**172.**	b	**192.**	d
133.	b	**153.**	c	**173.**	d	**193.**	c
134.	b	**154.**	a	**174.**	c	**194.**	d
135.	d	**155.**	b	**175.**	d	**195.**	a
136.	d	**156.**	a	**176.**	b	**196.**	c
137.	d	**157.**	a	**177.**	a	**197.**	b
138.	d	**158.**	c	**178.**	b	**198.**	a
139.	d	**159.**	b	**179.**	d	**199.**	a
140.	d	**160.**	a	**180.**	d	**200.**	a

7 Diseases of the Nervous System

Praveen Kumar and Sunil Punia

Introduction

The major components of the nervous system are the brain, the cranial nerves, the spinal cord and the peripheral nerves. The functions of the nervous system are directed at the maintenance of the body's spatial relationship with its environment. Abnormal mentation, involuntary movements, abnormal posture and gait, paresis or paralysis, blindness and altered sensation are the major clinical manifestations of nervous system disease. The manifestation of clinical signs depends on the location of the lesion within the nervous system. Abnormalities of mentation, posture, and gait are initially evaluated. Postural reactions are then evaluated. If abnormalities are detected, evaluation of muscle tone, spinal reflexes, urinary tract function and sensory perception aids in lesion localization. Finally, cranial nerves are evaluated, and if necessary, localization of a lesion within the brain is attempted. This will help in establishing an accurate neuroanatomic diagnosis. In addition to neurological examination, diagnostic techniques like cerebrospinal fluid (CSF) collection and analysis, radiography, computed tomography, magnetic resonance imaging, ophthalmoscopy, electroencephalography, etc., help in accurate neuroanatomic diagnosis of disease. CSF is collected from the cerebellomedullary cistern or the subarachnoid space in the lumbar region. Cell counts and identification should be performed within 30 minutes of collection. An increase in protein is often associated with encephalitis, meningitis, neoplasia or spinal cord compression. There are limitations in the neurological examination of large animals.

Altered mentation or seizures with a relatively normal gait are the most pronounced abnormalities in animals with forebrain disease, whereas dull mentation, proprioceptive ataxia and multiple cranial nerve deficits suggest brainstem disease. Hypermetria and ataxia are common in cerebellar disorders,

© CAB International 2024. *Key Questions in Clinical Farm Animal Medicine Volume 1: Principles of Disease Examination, Diagnosis and Management* (ed. T. Rana)
DOI: 10.1079/9781800624788.0007

and lesions of the central vestibular system within the brainstem or cerebellum usually cause a head tilt, loss of balance and nystagmus.

The clinical features of seizures can be separated into four components: prodrome, aura, ictal period and postictal period.Chronic management of dogs and cats with seizures can be attempted using anti-epileptic drugs like phenobarbital, potassium bromide, diazepam, levetiracetam, zonisamide, gabapentine, etc. Bacterial, viral, protozoal, mycotic, rickettsial and parasitic pathogens are all recognized as etiologic agents of infectious inflammatory central nervous system (CNS) disease in dogs and cats. Spinal cord disorders can be caused by anomalies, degeneration, neoplasia, inflammatory conditions, external trauma, internal trauma from disc extrusion, haemorrhage or infarction. Neoplasia and type II intervertebral disc (IVD) protrusion occur most commonly in middle-aged and older dogs.

Congenital malformations are present at birth, generally do not progress, and are often breed-associated. Type I disc extrusions primarily occur in chondrodystrophic small breeds of dogs. Functionally, the spinal cord can be divided into four regions: the cranial cervical spinal cord (C1–C5), cervical intumescence (C6–T2), thoracolumbar region (T3–L3) and lumbar intumescence (L4–S3). A lesion of the upper motor neuron causes spasticity with loss of voluntary movement, increased tone of limb muscles and increased spinal reflexes, while a lesion of the lower motor neuron causes paresis or paralysis with loss of voluntary movement, decreased tone of the limb muscles, absence of spinal reflexes and wasting of the affected muscle.

Multiple Choice Questions

1.   **Which of the following is not a component of the forebrain?**

   a. Cerebral cortex

   b. Thalamus

   c. Hypothalamus

   d. None of these

2.   **Appetite, thirst and body temperature are controlled by:**

   a. Hypothalamus

   b. Cerebrum

   c. Cerebellum

   d. Medulla oblongata

3.   **Intention tremor is associated with diseases of the:**

   a. Midbrain

   b. Medulla oblongata

   c. Cerebral cortex

   d. Cerebellum

4.   **Behaviour, vision, hearing and conscious perception of touch, pain, temperature and body position (proprioception) are associated with:**

   a. Midbrain

   b. Medulla oblongata

   c. Cerebral cortex

   d. Cerebellum

5.   **Frontal lobe lesion results in:**

   a. Blindness

   b. Voluntary motor function loss

   c. Disequilibrium

   d. Change in perception of pressure

6. **Occipital lobe lesion results in:**
   a. Blindness
   b. Seizures
   c. Disequilibrium
   d. Loss of memory

7. **Parietal lobe lesion results in:**
   a. Seizures
   b. Blindness
   c. Touch, pain, temperature misinterpretation
   d. Loss of memory

8. **Temporal lobe lesion causes:**
   a. Hypermetria
   b. Sound perception disability
   c. Balancing difficulty
   d. Nociception

9. **Central blindness is identified by:**
   a. Negative menace response
   b. Positive PLR
   c. a and b
   d. Negative PLR

10. **Peripheral blindness is identified by:**
    a. Positive menace response
    b. Negative PLR
    c. Positive PLR
    d. a and b

11. **Central blindness is associated with:**
    a. Retinal lesion
    b. PEM

c. Hypovitaminosis A

d. All of these

12. **Peripheral blindness is associated with:**

a. Retinal lesion

b. PEM

c. Occipital lobe lesion

d. a and c

13. **The ascending reticular activating system which regulates the consciousness is located in the:**

a. Pons and medulla

b. Cerebral cortex

c. Diencephalon

d. Cerebellum

14. **The normal respiratory regulating centre is present in the:**

a. Cerebellum

b. Cerebral cortex

c. Brain stem

d. Hypothalamus

15. **Head tilt, nystagmus and disequilibrium are due to lesion of:**

a. Vestibular system

b. Cerebral cortex

c. Diencephalon

d. Otitis

16. **Seizures are caused by lesion in the:**

a. Forebrain

b. Brainstem

c. Cerebellum

d. Thalamus

17. **Which of the following is false for forebrain lesion?**

    a. Postural reaction deficits in contralateral limbs

    b. Contralateral blindness with normal PLR

    c. Abnormal gait

    d. Altered mentation

18. **Wide-based stance, hypermetria, ataxia with normal strength and normal postural reactions are clinical signs resulting from lesion of:**

    a. Medulla oblongata

    b. Pons

    c. Cerebellum

    d. Limbic system

19. **Choose correct pairings:**

1. Myelencephalon	i) Cerebral cortex
2. Metencephalon	ii) Midbrain
3. Mesencephalon	iii) Medulla Oblongata
4. Diencephalon	iv) Pons
5. Telencephalon	v) Hypothalamus

    a. 1 – ii, 2 – i, 3 – v, 4 – iv, 5 – iii

    b. 1 – i, 2 – ii, 3 – iv, 4 – v, 5 – iii

    c. 1 – iv, 2 – i, 3 – ii, 4 – iii, 5 – v

    d. 1 – iii, 2 – iv, 3 – ii, 4 – v, 5 – i

20. **What is the name of the neuron that carries information from the peripheral nervous system to the central nervous system?**

    a. Afferent neuron

    b. Efferent neuron

    c. a and b

    d. Interneuron

21. **The peripheral nervous system (PNS) is formed by the:**

    a. Cranial nerves

    b. Spinal nerves

    c. a and b

    d. None of these

22. **Cauda equina lesion results in:**

    a. Atonic bladder

    b. Dilated and unresponsive anus

    c. Flaccid tail

    d. All of these

23. **Upper motor neurons are present in:**

    a. Brainstem and spinal cord

    b. Brainstem only

    c. Cerebrum only

    d. Cerebrum and brainstem

24. **Lower motor neuron cell bodies lie in the:**

    a. Brainstem and spinal cord

    b. Brainstem only

    c. Spinal cord only

    d. Cerebrum and brainstem

25. **Vestibular nuclei are present in the:**

    a. Cerebellum

    b. Brainstem

    c. a and b

    d. None of these

26. **Smell and emotional reactions are associated with the:**

    a. Paleocortex

    b. Archicortex

c. Neocortex

d. a and b

27. **What are best described as brief, intermittent titanic contractions of the skeletal muscles resulting in the entire body being rigid for several seconds, followed by relaxation?**

a. Fasciculations

b. Seizures

c. Tremors

d. Myoclonus

28. **What is best described as continuous, repetitive twitching of skeletal muscles that is usually visible and palpable?**

a. Tremors

b. Tics

c. Fasciculations

d. Convulsions

29. **What is best described as spasmodic twitching movements made at much longer intervals than in tremor?**

a. Tetany

b. Convulsions

c. Tics

d. Myoclonus

30. **What is best described as violent muscular contractions affecting part or all of the body and occurring for relatively short periods as a rule?**

a. Fits

b. Tetany

c. Tremors

d. All of these

31. **A menace response test is used to assess:**

    a. CN II and VII

    b. CN II and III

    c. CN II only

    d. CN III, IV and VI

32. **Pupillary light reflex evaluates:**

    a. CN II only

    b. CN II and III

    c. CN III, IV and VI

    d. CN III only

33. **Queckenstedt's test is used to determine or assess:**

    a. Thoracic and pelvic limb strength

    b. CSF pressure

    c. Protein in CSF

    d. Gastrocnemius spinal reflex

34. **Pleocytosis is the term used for:**

    a. Epithelial cells in CSF

    b. Increased pus cells in CSF

    c. Mitotic cells in CSF

    d. Macrophages in CSF

35. **Panniculus reflex is also known as:**

    a. Patellar reflex

    b. Perineal reflex

    c. Cutaneous trunci reflex

    d. Crossed extensor reflex

36. **A panniculus reflex test evaluates which spinal cord segment?**

    a. C1-C5

    b. C6-T2

c. C8-T1

d. L4-S3

37. Schiff-Sherrington posture evaluates which spinal cord segment?

a. C1-C5

b. C6-T2

c. T3-L1

d. L4-S3

38. With a spinal cord injury, what deficit causes 'knuckling' and a lack of awareness of where one's limbs are in space?

a. Sciatic nerve deficit

b. Conscious proprioceptive deficit

c. Menace reflect deficit

d. Autonomic receptive deficit

39. An oculo-cephalic response test evaluates:

a. CN VIII

b. CN III, IV, VI

c. CN III, IV, VI, VIII

d. CN III only

40. A palpebral reflex test evaluates:

a. CN V and VII

b. CN III, IV, VI

c. CN VII and VIII

d. CN II, III and IV

41. Gag reflex is used to evaluate:

a. Facial nerve

b. Vagus nerve

c. Trigeminal nerve

d. Hypoglossal nerve

42. **Tight circling toward the side of the lesion is often associated with:**

   a. Forebrain lesion

   b. Otitis media

   c. Vestibular disease

   d. None of these

43. **Ataxia can be caused by lesion of:**

   a. Cerebellum

   b. Vestibular system

   c. General proprioceptive (GP) sensory tracts in the spinal cord and caudal brainstem

   d. All of these

44. **Strabismus is:**

   a. Unequal size of pupils

   b. Abnormal movement of eyeball

   c. Abnormal position of eyeball

   d. Excessive lachrymation

45. **Oculomotor nerve dysfunction results in:**

   a. Medial strabismus

   b. Dorsolateral strabismus

   c. Ventrolateral strabismus

   d. Ventrodorsal strabismus

46. **Trochlear nerve dysfunction results in:**

   a. Dorsolateral strabismus

   b. Ventrolateral strabismus

   c. a and b

   d. None of these

47.   **Abducent nerve dysfunction results in:**

a. Medial strabismus

b. Lateral strabismus

c. Ventral strabismus

d. Dorsal strabismus

48.   **Animal jaw tone assessment is used in the evaluation of:**

a. CN VII

b. CN V

c. CN XII

d. All of these

49.   **Which cranial nerve is examined for head tilt?**

a. CN V

b. CN VII

c. CN VIII

d. CN IX

50.   **Anosmia is associated with:**

a. CN I

b. CN III

c. CN V

d. CN VII

51.   **Forebrain lesion in dogs causes:**

a. Blindness

b. Contralateral clinical signs

c. Seizure

d. All of these

52.   **The normal colour of CSF in horses is:**

a. Straw colour

b. White

c. Turbid

d. Colourless

53. **Menace response will be absent for how many days in calves?**

   a. 60

   b. 40

   c. 30

   d. 10

54. **Menace response will be absent for how many weeks in puppies?**

   a. 2–4

   b. 4–6

   c. 6–8

   d. 10–12

55. **Which of the following systems controls the activity in smooth and cardiac muscles and glands?**

   a. CNS

   b. PNS

   c. ANS

   d. CVS

56. **Cauda equine is associated with:**

   a. Thoracic limbs

   b. Pelvic limbs

   c. Bladder, anus and tail

   d. Head

57. **Spinal cord lesion from C1 to C5 can cause:**

   a. Spinal reflexes to remain intact in forelimbs and hindlimbs

   b. Tetraparesis

   c. Hemiparesis

   d. All of these

58. **Spinal cord lesion from C6 to T2 causes:**

    a. Depressed or absent spinal reflexes in forelimbs

    b. Tetraplegia

    c. Intact spinal reflexes in hindlimbs

    d. All of these

59. **Spinal cord lesion from L4 to S2 can cause:**

    a. Normal spinal reflexes in forelimbs

    b. Spinal reflexes absent or depressed in hindlimbs

    c. Conscious proprioceptive deficits and loss of perineal sensation

    d. All of these

60. **Spinal cord lesion from T3 to L3 causes:**

    a. Tetraparesis

    b. Hindlimb ataxia

    c. Forelimb ataxia

    d. Decreased spinal reflexes in forelimbs

61. **Spinal cord lesion from T3 to L3 are linked with:**

    a. Tetraparesis

    b. Pelvic limb ataxia

    c. Forelimbs and hindlimbs having intact spinal reflexes

    d. Conscious proprioceptive deficits

62. **Injury to the pons can result in:**

    a. Abnormal mentation

    b. Ipsilateral deficits

    c. CN V deficit

    d. All of these

63. **Vestibular nuclei are located in:**

    a. The medulla oblongata

    b. The cerebellum

c. a and b

d. None of these

64. **Which of the following cranial nerves doesn't originate from the brainstem?**

   a. CN I

   b. CN III

   c. CN V

   d. CN VII

65. **Contra-lateral clinical signs occur due to lesion of:**

   a. Forebrain

   b. Brainstem

   c. Cerebellum

   d. All of these

66. **In normal animals, the number of white blood cells per microlitre in CSF is:**

   a. > 50

   b. <5

   c. < 50

   d. > 5

67. **Moderate pleocytosis occurs when the WBC number in CSF is:**

   a. 5–10 cells/μL

   b. 6–49 cells/μL

   c. >200 cells/μL

   d. 50–200 cells/μL

68. **A Pandy's test is performed to examine the:**

   a. Blood

   b. Urine

   c. CSF

   d. Rumen fluid

69. **A Pandy's test is used to detect what in CSF?**

    a. Glucose

    b. Triglyceride

    c. White blood cells

    d. Protein

70. **The preferred site for CSF collection in cattle is:**

    a. Atlano-occipital cistern

    b. Thoracolumbar cistern

    c. Lumbosacral cistern

    d. Sacro-coccygeal cistern

71. **The site of choice for CSF collection in dogs is:**

    a. Atlano-occipital cistern

    b. Thoracolumbar cistern

    c. Lumbosacral cistern

    d. Sacro-coccygeal cistern

72. **The normal protein level in CSF collected from the cerebello-medullary cistern site in healthy dogs is:**

    a. <25 mg/dl

    b. <40 mg/dl

    c. <80 mg/dl

    d. <100 mg/dl

73. **The normal protein level in CSF collected from the lumbosacral cistern site in healthy dogs is:**

    a. <25 mg/dl

    b. <40 mg/dl

    c. <80 mg/dl

    d. <100 mg/dl

74. **The normal protein level in CSF collected from the lumbo-sacral cistern site in healthy cattle is:**

    a. <25 mg/dl

    b. <40 mg/dl

    c. <80 mg/dl

    d. <100 mg/dl

75. **The normal protein level in CSF collected from a healthy horse is:**

    a. <25 mg/dl

    b. <40 mg/dl

    c. <80 mg/dl

    d. <100 mg/dl

76. **Lateral deviation of the vertebral contour is known as:**

    a. Kyphosis

    b. Lordosis

    c. Scoliosis

    d. Swayback

77. **Dorsal deviation of the vertebral contour is known as:**

    a. Kyphosis

    b. Lordosis

    c. Scoliosis

    d. Swayback

78. **Ventral deviation of the vertebral contour is known as:**

    a. Kyphosis

    b. Lordosis

    c. Scoliosis

    d. None of these

79. **A 'wheelbarrowing' reaction detects dysfunction of which segment of the spinal cord?**

   a. Cervical

   b. Thoracic

   c. Lumbar

   d. Sacral

80. **Wheelbarrowing reaction is used to assess dysfunction of which body part of a dog?**

   a. Urinary bladder

   b. Thoracic limbs

   c. Eyes

   d. All of these

81. **Horner syndrome occurs due to:**

   a. Loss of sympathetic innervations to the eye

   b. Loss of parasympathetic innervations to the eye

   c. Loss of sympathetic innervations to the urinary bladder

   d. Loss of parasympathetic innervations to the urinary bladder

82. **Which of the following cranial nerves cannot be evaluated reliably in ruminants?**

   a. CN I

   b. CN XI

   c. a and b

   d. CN XII

83. **Which is the only postural reaction that can be evaluated in adult cattle?**

   a. Placing reaction

   b. Hopping

   c. Proprioception

   d. Wheelbarrowing

84. **In ruminants, which of the following spinal reflexes is not routinely evaluated?**

    a. Panniculus reflex

    b. Patellar reflex

    c. Withdrawal reflex

    d. Cranial tibial reflex

85. **The clinical state when animals tend to sleep if not disturbed and are unresponsive to environmental stimulation but responsive to noxious stimulus is:**

    a. Depression

    b. Coma

    c. Syncope

    d. Stupor

86. **An unconscious state in which an animal is unresponsive to noxious stimulus is:**

    a. Depression

    b. Coma

    c. Syncope

    d. Stupor

87. **Proprioception can be evaluated by:**

    a. Hopping

    b. Knuckling

    c. Placing reaction

    d. Wheelbarrowing

88. **Which of the following is not a postural reaction?**

    a. External postural thrust

    b. Placing

    c. Crossed extensor reflex

    d. Wheelbarrowing

89.   **Which of the following is not a spinal reflex?**

a. Babenski reflex

b. Patellar reflex

c. Perineal reflex

d. Knuckling

90.   **Which of the following is true regarding spinal reflexes?**

a. Help in classification of UMN versus LMN disorders

b. Mostly tested in lateral recumbency

c. Include myotatic and flexor reflexes

d. All of these

91.   **Which of the following is true for lower motor neurone disease?**

a. Flaccid paralysis

b. Muscle atrophy

c. Absence of spinal reflexes

d. All of these

92.   **Upper motor neurone disease causes:**

a. Spastic paralysis

b. Increased spinal reflexes

c. Increased tone of limb muscles

d. All of these

93.   **The most reliable spinal reflex tested routinely for pelvic limbs is:**

a. Cranial tibial reflex

b. Gastrocnemius reflex

c. a and b

d. Patellar reflex

94.   **Withdrawal reflex for thoracic limbs assesses:**

a. C6–T2 spinal cord segment

b. Nerves of brachial plexus

c. C1–C5 segment

d. a and b

95. **Withdrawal reflex for pelvic limbs assesses:**

a. L6–S1 spinal cord segment

b. Sciatic nerve

c. Only femoral nerve

d. a and b

96. **Which of the following tests should be carried out to assess the sciatic nerve?**

a. Patellar reflex

b. Cranial tibial reflex

c. Gastrocnemius reflex

d. b and c

97. **In dogs, abnormal bilateral patellar reflex suggests which-neuroanatomical location of lesion?**

a. L4–L6 spinal cord segment

b. L6–S1 spinal cord segment

c. S1–S3 spinal cord segment

d. a and b

98. **Femoral nerve injury can be assessed in/by:**

a. Lateral recumbency

b. Stifle extension on striking plexor

c. Patellar reflex

d. All of these

99. **Which of the following spinal reflexes is most difficult to elicit in normal dogs?**

a. Patellar reflex

b. Biceps and triceps reflex

    c. Crossed extensor reflex

    d. Withdrawal reflex

100. **Pudendal nerve and sacral spinal cord segments (S1–S3) are assessed by:**

    a. Perineal reflex

    b. Panniculus reflex

    c. Patellar reflex

    d. Proprioception

101. **Fluid in T1-weighted images of MRI appears as:**

    a. Grey

    b. White

    c. Black

    d. Red

102. **Short tau inversion recovery (STIR) sequence or fluid attenuated inversion recovery (FLAIR) sequence are used in which imaging modality?**

    a. MRI

    b. Electroencephalography

    c. Electromyography

    d. Computed tomography

103. **Short tau inversion recovery (STIR) sequence in MRI has been designed to suppress the signal from:**

    a. Fluid

    b. Fat

    c. Bone

    d. All of these

104. **'Actual seizure' is called the:**

    a. Prodromal period

    b. Aura

    c. Ictus

    d. Post-ictal period

105. **What is the name for the stereotypic motor, behavioural or autonomic changes that occur seconds to minutes before ictus?**

    a. Prodromal period

    b. Aura

    c. Ictus

    d. Post-ictus

106. **Which of these is a disorder of the brain marked by sudden recurring attacks of excessive sleep?**

    a. Obtundation

    b. Epilepsy

    c. Encephalomalacia

    d. Narcolepsy

107. **Continuous seizure activity lasting 5 minutes or longer without periods of intervening consciousness is called:**

    a. Cataplexy

    b. Convulsions

    c. Status epilepticus

    d. Epileptogenesis

108. **The first choice anti-epileptic drug for cats is:**

    a. Diazepam

    b. Potassium bromide

    c. Phenobarbital

    d. Levitiracetam

109. **The most life-threatening potential complication of chronic phenobarbital therapy is:**

    a. Nephrotoxicity

    b. Hepatotoxicity

c. Ototoxicity

d. Bone marrow toxicity

110. **Which of the following is a sign of increased intracranial pressure?**

a. Decreased arterial blood pressure

b. Altered breathing pattern

c. Abnormal behaviour

d. Bradycardia

111. **Potassium bromide is contraindicated in cats because it can cause:**

a. Hepatotoxicity

b. Nephrotoxicity

c. Bronchitis

d. All of these

112. **The starting dose of KBr when used as an add-on drug to phenobarbital is:**

a. 20 mg/kg orally twice daily

b. 15 mg/kg orally twice daily

c. 10 mg/kg orally twice daily

d. 2 mg/kg orally twice daily

113. **An appropriate starting dose of phenobarbital is:**

a. 2.5–3 mg/kg orally twice a day

b. 5.5–10 mg/kg orally twice a day

c. 10–15 mg/kg orally twice a day

d. 1–2.5 mg/kg orally twice a day

114. **Which anti-epileptic drug should not be prescribed to patients with a history of sulfonamide drug hypersensitivity?**

a. Zonisamide

b. Gabapentin

c. Diazepam

d. Levetiracetam

115. **Which anti-epileptic drug is not usually recommended for therapeutic monitoring?**

a. Diazepam

b. Zonisamide

c. Pheobarbital

d. Levetiracetam

116. **'At-home' injectable diazepam preparation can be administered in what way at onset of cluster seizures?**

a. Intramuscularly

b. Subcutaneously

c. Rectally

d. Intradermally

117. **What are the clinical signs of peripheral vestibular disease?**

a. Verticle nystagmus

b. Depression

c. Otitis + CN VII deficit

d. Abnormal postural reaction

118. **Multiple cranial nerve deficits indicate lesion present in the:**

a. Forebrain

b. Midbrain

c. Hindbrain

d. Spinal cord

119. **What are the clinical signs of central vestibular disease?**

a. Horizontal nystagmus

b. Multiple cranial nerve deficit

c. Normal proprioception

d. All of these

120. **Which of the following diseases can cause peripheral vestibular disease?**

    a. Otitis media-interna

    b. Aminoglycoside toxicity

    c. Trauma to petrous temporal bone

    d. All of these

121. **Verticle nystagmus can be found in:**

    a. Canine distemper

    b. Thiamine deficiency

    c. Meningioma

    d. All of these

122. **The most common cause of seizure in dogs is:**

    a. Intracranial

    b. Extracranial

    c. Idiopathic

    d. Metabolic

123. **The interictal period in idiopathic epilepsy is:**

    a. > 4 hours

    b. > 4 days

    c. > 4 weeks

    d. > 4 months

124. **Reactive seizures are caused by:**

    a. Intracranial disease

    b. Extracranial disease

    c. a and b

    d. None of these

125. **Which of the following is true for Type I IVDD in dogs?**

    a. Most common in aging large-breed non-chondrodystrophic dogs

    b. Results in slow progressive spinal cord compression

c. Thoracolumbar IVDD is more common than cervical IVDD

d. All of these

126. **Type II IVD is most common in which breed of dog?**

a. Dachshund

b. Beagle

c. Shih Tzu

d. German shepherd

127. **Thoracolumbar IVD extrusions are most common in:**

a. Dachshunds

b. Beagles

c. Labrador retrievers

d. Rottweilers

128. **Persistent ventroflexion of the neck is characteristic of:**

a. Hypokalaemia

b. Hyperkalaemia

c. Hypernatremia

d. Hyponatremia

129. **Opisthotonos results in:**

a. Ventroflexion of neck and flexor rigidity of limbs

b. Dorsiflexion of neck and flexor rigidity of limbs

c. Ventroflexion of neck and extensor rigidity of limbs

d. Dorsiflexion of neck and extensor rigidity of limbs

130. **Dyskinesias are related to:**

a. Voluntary movements

b. Involuntary movements

c. a and b

d. None of these

131.   **Femoral nerve lesion results in:**

   a. Animal unable to support its weight

   b. Inability to extend stifle and atrophy of quadriceps

   c. Loss of patellar reflex

   d. All of these

132.   **Lesion of the radial nerve causes:**

   a. Reduced extension of elbow

   b. Reduced flexion of elbow

   c. Loss of shoulder extension

   d. Reduced flexion of carpus

133.   **Plantigrade pelvic limb stance in cats is seen in which condition?**

   a. Diabetic polyneuropathy

   b. Chronic idiopathic demyelinating polyneuropathies

   c. Coonhound paralysis

   d. All of these

134.   **Coonhound paralysis is associated with:**

   a. Myasthenia gravis

   b. Tick paralysis

   c. Acute polyradiculoneuritis

   d. All of these

135.   **Which of the following is not associated with acute poly-radiculoneuritis?**

   a. Normal cranial nerves

   b. Hyperaesthesia

   c. Rapid progressive muscle atrophy

   d. None of these

136. **Rapidly progressive lower motor neurone tetraparesis in dogs is caused by:**

   a. Coonhound paralysis

   b. Tick paralysis

   c. Myasthenia gravis

   d. All of these

137. **Which clinical sign differentiates acute polyradiculoneuritis from tick paralysis?**

   a. Normal cranial nerves

   b. Decreased muscle tone

   c. Hyperaesthesia

   d. a and b

138. **Which peripheral nerve is affected in curled toe paralysis of chickens?**

   a. Tibial

   b. Femoral

   c. Radial

   d. Sciatic

139. **The most severe form of injury to the peripheral nerve is:**

   a. Neuropraxia

   b. Axonotmesis

   c. Neurotmesis

   d. None of these

140. **Myelitis is inflammation of:**

   a. Muscles

   b. Intervertebral discs

   c. Mylencephalon

   d. Spinal cord

141. **The most common tumour of the spinal cord is:**

    a. Meningiomas

    b. Osteosarcoma

    c. Peripheral nerve sheath

    d. All of these

142. **'Wobbler syndrome' is the term used for:**

    a. Polyradiculoneuritis

    b. Intervertebral disc disease

    c. Discospondylitis

    d. Cervical spondylomyelopathy

143. **Schiff-Sherrington phenomenon indicates injury to the:**

    a. Cervical spinal cord

    b. Brainstem

    c. Forebrain

    d. Thoracolumbar spinal cord

144. **In canine distemper, neurological signs are due to:**

    a. Encephalitis

    b. Myelitis

    c. Encephalomyelitis

    d. None of these

145. **Anisocoria is:**

    a. Loss of vision

    b. Unequal vision

    c. Abnormal eyeball position

    d. Unequal pupil size

146. **Which of these is not a symptom of Horner syndrome?**

    a. Prolapsed nictitans

    b. Drooping of upper eyelids

    c. Dilatation of pupils

    d. Inward sinking of eyeballs

147. **Constant myoclonus occurs secondarily due to:**

    a. Tetanus

    b. Mg deficiency

    c. Ca deficiency

    d. Canine distemper

148. **Softening of grey matter in the brain is known as:**

    a. Leukoencephalomalacia

    b. Polioencephalomalacia

    c. Myelomalacia

    d. None of these

149. **In cattle, a common cause of meningitis or encephalitis is:**

    a. Viruses

    b. Parasite migration

    c. Fungi

    d. Bacteria

150. **In horses and dogs, meningitis or encephalitis occurs more frequently due to:**

    a. Bacteria

    b. Viruses

    c. Parasites

    d. All of these

151. **Which mycoplasma causes encephalitis in goats?**

    a. *M.mycoides*

    b. *M. edwardii*

    c. *M. pulmonis*

    d. *M. bovis*

152. The predilection site for lesion caused by listeriosis is:

a. Lumbar intumescence

b. Cerebrum

c. Brainstem

d. Cervical intumescence

153. Which of the following viruses is in the main spread trans-axonally to CNS?

a. Morbillivirus

b. Parvovirus

c. Herpesvirus

d. Rabies

154. Which of the following fungi can cause meningoencephalitis?

a. *Coccidioides immitis*

b. *Blastomyces dermatitidis*

c. *Histoplasma capsulatum*

d. All of these

155. Which of the following protozoa can cause meningoencephalitis in dogs?

a. *Dirofilaria immitis*

b. *Trypanosoma* spp.

c. *Sarcocystis neurona*

d. *Toxoplasma gondii*

156. Trigeminal and facial nerve paralysis occurs in:

a. Listeriosis

b. PEM

c. Chiari-like malformations

d. All of these

157. **Polioencephalomalacia (PEM) is an important neurological disease of which species?**

a. Horses

b. Dogs

c. Pigs

d. Cattle

158. **Which disease of sheep is also known as ovine encephalo-myelitis?**

a. Scrapie

b. Louping III

c. PEM

d. Pregnancy toxaemia

159. **Important clinical signs of meningitis are:**

a. Fever

b. Hyperesthesia

c. Neck rigidity

d. All of these

160. **Chiari-like malformations are associated with:**

a. Cerebellar infarction

b. Cerebellar inflammation

c. Cerebellar tumour

d. Metronidazole toxicity

161. **Development of a CSF-filled cavity (syrinx) within the paren-chyma of the spinal cord is known as:**

a. Hydromyelia

b. Synringomyelia

c. Wobbler syndrome

d. Spina bifida

162. **Chiari-like malformations are associated with:**

    a. Back pain

    b. Neck pain

    c. Thoracic pain

    d. Pelvic pain

163. **Degenerative disorders of the nervous system are characterized as:**

    a. Per acute

    b. Subacute progressive

    c. Chronic progressive

    d. All of these

164. **Infectious and noninfectious inflammatory disease of the spinal cord falls into which category?**

    a. Per acute

    b. Subacute progressive

    c. Chronic progressive

    d. All of these

165. **The preferred imaging modality for assessment of most neurological problems is:**

    a. MRI

    b. Computed tomography

    c. Electroencephalography

    d. Radiography

166. **Bony lesions in diseases of the nervous system are best imaged using:**

    a. MRI

    b. Computed tomography

    c. Electroencephalography

    d. Radiography

167. **Fluid in T2-weighted images of MRI appears as:**

   a. Grey

   b. White

   c. Black

   d. Red

Answers

1.	d	31.	a	61.	a	91.	d
2.	a	32.	b	62.	d	92.	d
3.	d	33.	b	63.	c	93.	d
4.	c	34.	b	64.	a	94.	d
5.	b	35.	c	65.	a	95.	d
6.	a	36.	c	66.	b	96.	d
7.	c	37.	c	67.	d	97.	a
8.	b	38.	b	68.	c	98.	d
9.	c	39.	c	69.	d	99.	b
10.	b	40.	a	70.	c	100.	a
11.	b	41.	b	71.	a	101.	b
12.	a	42.	c	72.	a	102.	a
13.	a	43.	d	73.	b	103.	b
14.	c	44.	c	74.	b	104.	c
15.	a	45.	d	75.	d	105.	b
16.	a	46.	a	76.	c	106.	d
17.	c	47.	a	77.	a	107.	c
18.	c	48.	b	78.	b	108.	c
19.	d	49.	c	79.	a	109.	b
20.	a	50.	a	80.	b	110.	d
21.	c	51.	d	81.	a	111.	c
22.	d	52.	d	82.	c	112.	b
23.	d	53.	d	83.	c	113.	a
24.	a	54.	d	84.	d	114.	a
25.	c	55.	c	85.	d	115.	d
26.	a	56.	c	86.	b	116.	c
27.	d	57.	d	87.	b	117.	c
28.	a	58.	d	88.	c	118.	c
29.	c	59.	d	89.	d	119.	b
30.	a	60.	b	90.	d	120.	d

(Continued)

121.	d	133.	a	145.	d	157.	d
122.	c	134.	c	146.	c	158.	b
123.	c	135.	d	147.	d	159.	d
124.	b	136.	d	148.	b	160.	a
125.	c	137.	c	149.	d	161.	b
126.	d	138.	d	150.	d	162.	b
127.	a	139.	c	151.	a	163.	c
128.	a	140.	d	152.	c	164.	b
129.	d	141.	b	153.	d	165.	a
130.	b	142.	d	154.	d	166.	b
131.	d	143.	d	155.	d	167.	c
132.	a	144.	c	156.	a		

8 Diseases of the Digestive System

Anil Kumar, Ankesh Kumar and Sonam Bhatt

Introduction

Gastrointestinal diseases constitute a major proportion of diseases in farm animals. The application of the physiology of characteristic reticulo-rumen motility can enhance the diagnosis, prognosis and treatment of stomach-related disorders. There are four major modes of alimentary dysfunction: abnormality of motility, secretion, digestion or absorption. The most frequent cause of gastrointestinal tract disease is abnormalities of the stomach and intestinal motility. The following can happen when the gastrointestinal tract's motility is disturbed:

- dehydration and stress
- hyper- or hypomotility
- tract segment distension
- abdominal pain

One of the main effects of abnormal motility is the distension of one or more gastrointestinal tract segments. The distension can be caused by accumulation of gas or fluid, or ingesta. Saliva, gastric and intestinal juices are normally released during normal digestion. Gases are produced by either regular digestive processes or aberrant fermentation and if not expelled normally (eructation or flatulence) lead to gas distension. The distension can lead to pain and, reflexively, increased spasm and motility of adjoining gut segments. The distension also further stimulates the secretion of fluid into the lumen of the intestine, and this exaggerates the distension. When the distension reaches a certain threshold, the wall's musculature loses its capacity, and the response diminishes. The initial pain disappears, and a state of paralytic ileus develops in which much muscle tone is lost. In ruminants, reticulo rumen motility is of major importance in the forestomach, and

© CAB International 2024. *Key Questions in Clinical Farm Animal Medicine Volume 1: Principles of Disease Examination, Diagnosis and Management* (ed. T. Rana)
DOI: 10.1079/9781800624788.0008

prehension, mastication and swallowing are also important in the alimentary tract motility that is essential for normal function. Eructation of ruminal gases is an additional important function of motility in ruminants.

The most important mechanism of abdominal (visceral) pain is stretching of the wall of the viscus, and stimulating free pain endings of nerves in the wall. Vomiting is typically classified as either peripheral or central in origin depending on whether the stimulation for vomiting arises centrally at the vomiting centre, peripherally from overloading the stomach, from inflammation of the gastric mucosa or from the presence of foreign bodies in the pharynx, oesophagus or oesophageal groove. True vomiting is not a feature of gastric disease in horses due to a strong cardiac sphincter and anatomical conformation of the soft palate. In horses, the stomach contents are discharged only through the nasal cavities. Dynamic or mechanical ileus is a state of physical obstruction. Impaction of the large intestine of horses is a form of ileus.

Multiple Choice Questions

1. **Complete atony and gross distension of the rumen are characteristics of:**

    a. Vagal Indigestion

    b. LDA

    c. RDA

    d. None of these

2. **Ping, a high-pitched metallic tympanic sound percussed and auscultated at the midpoint of the 9th to 13th rib of the left abdomen occurs in:**

    a. LDA

    b. Atonicrumen

    c. Pneumo-peritoneum

    d. All of these

3. **Biphasic contraction of the reticulum occurs in:**

    a. Primary cycle

    b. Secondary cycle

    c. a and b

    d. None of these

4. **In reticulo-rumen motility, the primary cycle is:**

    a. Eructation cycle

    b. Mixing cycle

    c. a and b

    d. None of these

5. **A 'papple'-shaped abdomen is observed in:**

    a. RDA

    b. LDA

    c. Vagal indigestion

    d. All of these

6. In the secondary cycle, the movement of the reticulo-rumen is confined to:

    a. Reticulum

    b. Dorsal sac of rumen

    c. Ventral sac of rumen

    d. b and c

7. An L-shaped rumen on rectal palpation occurs commonly in:

    a. Vegas indigestion

    b. RDA

    c. LDA

    d. All of these

8. A fluid splashing sound is commonly heard in:

    a. Grain overload

    b. Peritonitis

    c. Omasal/abomasal impaction

    d. All of these

9. Watery rumen content indicates what?

    a. Inactive bacteria

    b. Inactive protozoa

    c. Active protozoa

    d. a and b

10. The normal pH of rumen fluid is:

    a. 6.2–7.2

    b. 5.2–7.2

    c. 6.7–8.2

    d. All of these

11. High pH of rumen occurs in:

    a. Putrefaction of protein

    b. Putrefaction of carbohydrate

   c. Putrefaction of fatty acids

   d. All of these

12. Low pH of rumen occurs as a result of:

   a. Feeding of carbohydrate

   b. Feeding of protein

   c. Feeding of hay

   d. All of these

13. In carbohydrate engorgement, the pH range of rumen fluid is:

   a. Below 5

   b. Between 6.2–7.2

   c. Above 5

   d. All of these

14. In grain overload, examination of rumen fluid shows:

   a. Absence of protozoan

   b. Predominant gm +ve bacteria

   c. a and b

   d. None of these

15. Closure of the oesophageal groove in cattle can be induced by:

   a. Solute of NaCl

   b. Solute of sodium bicarbonate

   c. Sugar

   d. All of these

16. The following concentration of sodium bicarbonate induces oesophageal closure in cattle:

   a. 20% $NaHCO_3$

   b. 10% $NaHCO_3$

   c. 15% $NaHCO_3$

   d. None of these

17. **In adult cows, the reticulo-rumen has the capacity to hold:**

a. 70 kg of digests

b. 90 kg of digests

c. 80 kg of digests

d. None of these

18. **Buccal receptors are:**

a. Mechanoreceptors

b. Chemoreceptors

c. Thermoreceptors

d. All of these

19. **Which of the following is not a rumenotoric agent?**

a. Nux vomica

b. Ginger

c. Gentian

d. Belladonna

20. **The faeces of cows with LDA commonly appear:**

a. Pasty

b. Hard

c. Semi-solid

d. All of these

21. **The presence of a plug of mucus in the rectum is suggestive of:**

a. Physical obstruction

b. Functional obstruction

c. a and b

d. None of these

22. **The following agents are used to treat rumen alkalosis:**

 a. Acetic acid

 b. Vinegar

 c. a and b

 d. None of these

23. **Systemic acidosis is treated with an IV solution of:**

 a. 5% $NacHO_3$

 b. 10% $NaHCO_3$

 c. 2.5% $NaHCO_3$

 d. All of these

24. **Which of the following alkalinizing agents is used to treat acidosis?**

 a. $Mg(OH)_2$

 b. MgO

 c. a and b

 d. None of these

25. **Which of the following agents is used to prevent ruminal acidosis?**

 a. Salinomycin

 b. Monensin

 c. Lasalocid

 d. All of these

26. **Non-bloating forages prevent bloat due to their containing:**

 a. Tannins

 b. Lignins

 c. Chloroplast

 d. All of these

27. **Inadequate coalescence of bubbles in ruminants can lead to:**

   a. Free gas bloat

   b. Frothy bloat

   c. a and b

   d. None of these

28. **Mineral oil as an antifoaming agent is used to:**

   a. Increase surface tension

   b. Reduce surface tension

   c. a and b

   d. None of these

29. **Which of the following is an anti-foaming agent?**

   a. Poloxalene

   b. Sodium sulfosuccinate

   c. Mineral oil

   d. All of these

30. **Which of following is best used to treat leguminous bloat?**

   a. Poloxalehe

   b. Mineral oil

   c. a and b

   d. None of these

31. **Which of the following in not recommended to treat feedlot bloat?**

   a. Poloxalene

   b. Mineral oil

   c. a and b

   d. None of these

32. **To prevent leguminous bloat, the daily recommended dose of poloxalene is:**

   a. 2 g/100 kg

   b. 4 gm/100 kg

   c. 6 gm/ 100 kg

   d. All of these

33. **The recommended dose of poloxalene to treat leguminous bloat is:**

   a. 25–50 gm

   b. 50–100gm

   c. 10–25gm

   d. All of these

34. **Degenerative left shift occurs in:**

   a. Acute diffuse peritonitis

   b. Acute local peritonitis

   c. a and b

   d. None of these

35. **Regenerative left shift occurs in:**

   a. Acute local peritonitis

   b. Acute diffuse peritonitis

   c. a and b

   d. None of these

36. **Jaundice without impairment of bile flow is associated with:**

   a. Hepatitis

   b. Cholestasis

   c. Haemolytic jaundice

   d. All of these

37. **Hoflund syndrome is associated with:**

    a. Vagal indigestion

    b. Acidosis

    c. Tympany

    d. None of these

38. **Dorsal vagal nerve injury in cattle causes:**

    a. Anterior stenosis

    b. Posterior stenosis

    c. a and b

    b. None of these

39. **Dorsal and ventral vagal nerve injury in cattle leads to:**

    a. Scant faeces

    b. Undigested long feed particles

    c. a and b

    d. None of these

40. **Vagal indigestion in caused by**

    a. TRP

    b. Actinbacillosis of the rumen

    c. Reticular adhesion

    d. All of these

41. **Vagal indigestion is associated with:**

    a. Pyloric achalasia

    b. Late pregnancy

    c. Fibro papilloma at the cardia

    d. All of these

42. **Vagal indigestion can lead to metabolic:**

    a. Hypochloremic hypokalaemic alkalosis

    b. Hyperchloremic hypokalaemic alkalosis

c. a and b

d. None of these

43. **In cattle, the point of maximum heart sound can be auscultated in:**

    a. 4–5 intercostal space on the left side

    b. 4–5 intercostal space on the right side

    c. 3–4 intercostal space on the left side

    d. All of these

44. **Foul-smelling and turbid pericardial fluid indicates:**

    a. Peritonitis

    b. Pericarditis

    c. Ascites

    d. All of these

45. **In TRP, heart sounds are:**

    a. Muffled with fluid splashing sounds

    b. High-pitched gurgling sounds

    c. Low-pitched gurgling sounds

    d. All of these

46. **Ruminal sounds are usually not audible in:**

    a. Acidosis

    b. Vagal Indigestion

    c. Impaction

    d. Any of these

47. **LDA is mostly associated with:**

    a. Adequate level roughage

    b. Diet high in carbohydrate

    c. Adequate crude fibre

    d. All of these

48. **A slab-sided appearance of the left lateral abdomen occurs in:**

   a. Acidosis

   b. Impaction of rumen

   c. LDA

   d. None of these

49. **Which of the following is a common complication of LDA?**

   a. Acidosis

   b. Ketosis

   c. Impaction

   d. Ruminal atony

50. **Which of the following is a popular method of LDA correction?**

   a. Right paralumbar fossa omentopexy

   b. Right paramedian abomasopexy

   c. a and b

   d. None of these

51. **LDA can best be controlled by:**

   a. Avoiding negative energy balance

   b. Avoiding over-conditioning

   c. Maximizing dry matter intake

   d. All of these

52. **The most common aetiological factor of RDA is:**

   a. Abomasalatony

   b. Abomasal volvulus

   c. a and b

   d. None of these

53. **Caecal dilatation in cattle is effectively treated with:**

   a. Bethanecol

   b. Xylazine

c. a and b

d. None of these

54. **Lactose causes diarrhoea through a:**

a. Hypo-osmotic effect

b. Hyper-osmotic effect

c. Iso-osmotic effect

d. All of these

55. **The act of 'grasping of food' in cows is known as:**

a. Mastication

b. Prehension

c. Deglutination

d. All of these

56. **Swallowing is a complex act governed by reflexes and mediated through the:**

a. Pharyngeal nerve

b. Trigeminal nerve

c. Hypoglossal nerve

d. All of these

57. **Difficulty in swallowing is called:**

a. Dysphagia

b. Anophagia

c. Trichophagia

d. All of these

58. **Which of the following causes systemic excessive salivation?**

a. Iodism

b. Oral ulcers

c. Oesophageal abnormality

d. All of these

59. **Vomition involves:**

   a. Hypersalivation

   b. Retching

   c. Contraction of abdominal muscles and diaphragm

   d. All of these

60. **Psyllium mucilloid is the treatment of choice for:**

   a. Sand colic

   b. Spasmodic colic

   c. Flatulent colic

   d. All of these

61. **Projectile vomition is not accompanied by:**

   a. Retching

   b. Hypersalivation

   c. Forceful contraction of the abdomen

   d. All of these

62. **True vomition rarely occurs in**

   a. Farm animals

   b. Companion animals

   c. a and b

   d. None of these

63. **The vomition of large quantities of material in horses suggests:**

   a. Gastric torsion

   b. Gastric rupture

   c. Gastric volvulus

   d. All of these

64. **The expulsion of food material which has not yet reached the stomach is called:**

   a. Regurgitation

   b. Vomiting

c. a and b

d. None of these

65. **In cattle, regurgitation of large quantities of rumen content through the mouth occurs due to:**

a. Third-stage milk fever

b. Loss of cardia tone

c. Lamination of the cardia

d. All of these

66. **Vomition in pigs occurs due to:**

a. Transmissible gastroenteritis

b. *Fusarium* spp.

c. Acute chemical intoxication

d. All of these

67. **Faeces containing increased concentrations of water and reduced dry water content is known as:**

a. Diarrhoea

b. Constipation

c. Dysentery

d. None of these

68. **A decrease in the frequency of defecation is called:**

a. Constipation

b. Dysentery

c. Diarrhoea

d. All of these

69. **Scant faeces occurs most commonly in cattle with abnormalities of the:**

a. Fore stomach

b. Small intestine

c. Large intestine

d. All of these

70. **Dynamic ileus is a state of:**
    a. Functional obstruction
    b. Physical obstruction
    c. a and b
    d. None of these

71. **In grain overload, the colour of rumen juice appears as:**
    a. Milky-grey
    b. Yellow/bran
    c. Greenish-black
    d. None of these

72. **Mouldy, rotting rumen fluid indicates:**
    a. Protein putrefaction
    b. Carbohydrate putrefaction
    c. Fat indigestion
    d. All of these

73. **The normal pH range for rumen fluid is:**
    a. 6.2–7.2
    b. 7.2–8.2
    c. 6.8–8.2
    d. All of these

74. **Normal peritoneal fluid looks:**
    a. Straw-coloured to yellow
    b. Turbid
    c. Trans-opaque
    d. All of these

75. **Turbidity of peritoneal fluid indicates:**
    a. Increased leucocytes
    b. Increased protein

c. a and b

d. None of these

76. **An orange-green colour of peritoneal fluid indicates:**

a. Rupture of biliary system

b. Leakage of food materials

c. Leakage of intestine

d. All of these

77. **High specific gravity and high protein content of peritoneal fluid are indicative of:**

a. Peritonitis

b. Mural infarction

c. a and b

d. None of these

78 **An increase in the number of mesothelial cells in peritoneal fluid in cattle indicates:**

a. Neoplasia

b. Acute inflammation

c. Chronic inflammation

d. All of these

79. **In cattle, metoclopramide is indicated in:**

a. Reflux oesophagitis

b. Gastritis

c. Postoperative ileus

d. All of these

80. **In cattle, the correct dose of metoclopramide for rumen hypo-motility is:**

a. 0.3 mg/kg

b. 0.8 mg/kg

c. 1.1 mg/kg

d. 2.2 mg/kg

81. **Which of the following is used to reduce abdominal pain?**

a. Metoclopramide

b. Cisapride

c. Xylazine

d. Naloxone

82. **Which of the following is used to increase gastrointestinal motility?**

a. Cisapride

b. Metoclopramide

c. a and b

d. Atropine

83. **Inflammation of the oral mucosa is called:**

a. Stomatitis

b. Glossitis

c. Lampas

d. Palatitis

84. **Inflammation of the soft palate is called:**

a. Lampas

b. Glossitis

c. Gingivitis

d. None of these

85. **Bullous stomatitis occurs in:**

a. Horses

b. Cattle

c. Sheep

d. Goat

86. **Inflammation of the salivary gland is known as:**

    a. Parotitis

    b. Gingivitis

    c. Lampas

    d. Glossitis

87. **In pharyngitis, which of the following is not clinically characterized?**

    a. Coughing

    b. Painful swallowing

    c. Regurgitation

    d. Tympany

88. **Which of the following in not manifested in pharyngeal paralysis?**

    a. Inability to swallow

    b. Absence of signs of pain

    c. Respiratory obstruction

    d. Stertorous respiration

89. **Pharyngeal paralysis is not associated with:**

    a. Rabies

    b. Botulinum

    c. African horse sickness

    d. Pharyngeal cyst

90. **Cud droppings occur due to**

    a. Pharyngeal paralysis

    b. Pharyngeal obstruction

    c. Pharyngitis

    d. None of these

91. **Roaring is associated with:**

   a. Laryngeal paralysis

   b. Pharyngeal paralysis

   c. a and b

   d. None of these

92. **In horses, choke and drooling occur through the:**

   a. Nostrils

   b. Mouth

   c. a and b

   d. None of these

93. **Dilatation along the body of the oesophagus occurs in:**

   a. Megaoesophagus

   b. Oesophageal obstruction

   c. Oesophageal paralysis

   d. None of these

94. **The most common complication of megaoesophagus is:**

   a. Aspiration pneumonia

   b. Tympany

   c. Inability to eructate

   d. None of these

95. **The dose of phenylbutazone in equine colic is:**

   a. 8–10 mg/kg

   b. 2–4 mg/kg

   c. 0.5–2 mg/kg

   d. None of these

96. **Oesophageal relaxation, analgesia and anti-inflammatory effects are achieved by:**

   a. Hyoscine and dipyrone

   b. Xylazine and romfidine

    c. Xylazine and acepromazine

    d. None of these

97. **Which of the following is a frequent and important cause of death in horses?**

    a. Colic

    b. Impaction of colon

    c. Enteritis

    d. None of these

98. **Which of the following breeds of horse is at risk of colic?**

    a. Arabian horses

    b. Kathiwari horses

    c. a and b

    d. None of these

99. **There is less likelihood of colic:**

    a. Where horses are stabled

    b. Where horses are at pasture

    c. Where there is inconsistent access to water

    d. None of these

100. **In horses, the hallmark of gastrointestinal disease is:**

    a. Enteritis

    b. Pain

    c. Diarrhoea

    d. None of these

101. **In equines, pawing, stamping or kicking at the belly is suggestive of:**

    a. Enteritis in the intestine

    b. Flatulence in the abdomen

    c. Pain in the abdomen

    d. None of these

102. **Symmetrical severe distension of the abdomen in horses indicates:**

   a. Distention of the colon

   b. Distension of the caecum

   c. Distension of the intestine

   d. None of these

103. **Horses with a heart rate of more than 120 beats/minute are likely to be suffering from:**

   a. Mild disease

   b. Severe disease

   c. Moderate disease

   d. None of these

104. **Which of the following is a common clinical sign of abdominal pain in horses?**

   a. Sweating

   b. Bloating

   c. Grinding of teeth

   d. None of these

105. **Hyperkalaemia in equines is commonly associated with:**

   a. Acidosis

   b. Alkalosis

   c. Impaction of large colon

   d. None of these

106. **Horses with severe colic are likely to be suffering from:**

   a. Metabolic alkalosis

   b. Metabolic acidosis

   c. a and b

   d. None of these

107. **Plasma lactate concentration can be obtained by calculating:**

   a. Cation gap

   b. Anion gap

   c. Bicarbonate concentration

   d. None of these

108. **Elevated pulse rate with a fall in pulse amplitude is a reliable indicator of:**

   a. Dehydration

   b. Rehydration

   c. Shock

   d. a and c

109. **A small amplitude, thready pulse indicates:**

   a. Severe shock

   b. Mild shock

   c. Mild dehydration

   d. All of these

110. **A capillary refill time more than 2 seconds indicates:**

   a. Heart failure

   b. Peripheral circulatory failure

   c. Congestion

   d. None of these

111. **Which of the following analgesics is used in equine colic?**

   a. Flunixin meglumine

   b. Ketoprofen

   c. Phenylbutazone

   d. All of these

112. **Which of the following is an opiate used to treat colic in horses?**

   a. Butorphanol

   b. Xylazine

   c. Detomidine

   d. None of these

113. **Which of the following has a spasmolytic effect to treat colic in horses?**

   a. Atropine

   b. Hyoscine

   c. a and b

   d. None of these

114. **Which of the following has long-acting analgesic activity?**

   a. Flunixin meglumine

   b. Phenylbutazone

   c. Dipyrone

   d. None of these

115. **Which of the following can be used to treat mild cases of colic in equines?**

   a. Dipyrone

   b. Ketoprofen

   c. Flunixin meglumine

   d. None of these

116. **Which of the following is a pro-motility agent used to treat ileus or large colon impaction in equines?**

   a. Cisapride

   b. Psyllium

   c. Dioctyl sodium sulfosuccinate

   d. None of these

117.   **Which of the following is a faecal softener?**

   a. Magnesium sulfate

   b. Mineral oil

   c. Sodium bicarbonate

   d. None of these

118.   **In severe cases of flatulent colic in equines, trocarization is performed through the:**

   a. Left paralumbar fossa

   b. Right paralumbar fossa

   c. Ventral abdomen

   d. None of these

119.   **The following condition has a low survival rate in equines:**

   a. Lesions in the small intestine

   b. Lesions in the large intestine

   c. Non-strangulating diseases

   d. None of these

120.   **Meconium impaction is more common in:**

   a. Colt foals

   b. Fillies

   c. Adult horse

   d. None of these

121.   **Intussusceptions are most common in foals of what age?**

   a. 3–5 months

   b. 6 months

   c. 3 years

   d. None of these

122.   **Inguinal hernia occurs only in:**

   a. Female foals

   b. Male foals

   c. Miniature foals

   d. None of these

123. **Meconium impaction can be treated using:**

   a. Soap and water

   b. Acetyl cysteine

   c. Sodium bicarbonate

   d. All of these

124. **Which of the following is an ulcerogenic drug?**

   a. Phenylbutazone

   b. Xylazine

   c. Misoprostol

   d. None of these

125. **Which one of the following is an H_2 antagonist used to treat gastric ulcer in equines?**

   a. Cimetidine

   b. Omeprazole

   c. Sucralfate

   d. None of these

126. **Which one of the following is a gastrointestinal protectant?**

   a. Sucralfate

   b. Misoprostol

   c. Calcium carbonate

   d. None of these

127. **Omeprazole is a:**

   a. H_2 antagonist

   b. Proton pump inhibitor

   c. Protectant

   d. None of these

128. **Gastric ulcers in adult horses are associated with:**

   a. Parasitic gastritis

   b. Tumours of the gastric mucosa

   c. Phytobezoars

   d. All of these

129. **The dose of ranitidine to treat gastric ulcers in adult horses is:**

   a. 6.6 mg/kg

   b. 0.5 mg/kg

   c. 1 mg/kg

   d. None of these

130. **Which of the following is the most suitable for diagnosing small intestine obstruction?**

   a. Radiography

   b. Ultrasonography

   c. Endoscopy

   d. None of these

131. **Inguinal hernias occur only in:**

   a. Males

   b. Females

   c. a and b

   d. None of these

132. **Which one of the following diseases most commonly occurs in equines?**

   a. Caecal impaction

   b. Caecal rupture

   c. Caecal torsion

   d. None of these

133. **Volvulus is more commonly seen in:**

    a. Mares

    b. Stallions

    c. Foals

    d. None of these

134. **Which of the following acaricides causes impaction colic in horses?**

    a. Amitraz

    b. Deltamethrin

    c. Ivermectin

    d. None of these

135. **Most enteroliths in the large colon of horses are composed of:**

    a. Calcium oxalate

    b. Calcium carbonate

    c. Ammonium magnesium phosphate

    d. All of these

136. **Which of the following is a common colic type in horses?**

    a. Obstructive

    b. Spasmodic

    c. Flatulent

    d. All of these

137. **Verminus aneurysm in horses is caused by:**

    a. *Stongylus vulganis*

    b. *Cooperia punctata*

    c. *Dirofilaria immitis*

    d. All of these

138. **The presence of frank flood in faeces is called:**

    a. Melena

    b. Hematochezia

    c. Dysentery

    d. None of these

139. **In mature cattle, chronic diarrhoea with a history of chronic weight loss suggests:**

    a. Parasitic disease

    b. Johne's disease

    c. Dietary disease

    d. None of these

140. **Loperamide has one of the following effects:**

    a. Anti-secretary

    b. Intestinal protection

    c. Adsorbent

    d. None of these

141. **Prolapse of the rectum is most commonly seen in:**

    a. Pigs

    b. Cattle

    c. Horses

    d. None of these

142. **Which type of jaundice is the least intense?**

    a. Obstructive

    b. Hepatic

    c. a and b

    d. Haemolytic

143. **In haemolytic jaundice the urine contains:**

    a. Urobilinogen

    b. Bilirubin

c. a and b

d. None of these

144. **An increased level of bilirubin and urobilinogen in urine indicates:**

a. Hepatic jaundice

b. Haemolytic jaundice

c. Obstructive jaundice

d. All of these

145. **The presence of conjugated bilirubin in urine, but no urobilinogen, suggests:**

a. Hepatic jaundice

b. Haemolytic jaundice

c. Obstructive jaundice

d. All of these

146. **Examination of the liver of cattle is performed with:**

a. 3.5 MHz linear transducer

b. 7.5 MHz linear transducer

c. 8.5 MHz linear transducer

d. 5.5 MHz linear transducer

147. **Which of the following in not considered a sensitive indicator of hepatocellular injury?**

a. GGT

b. SDH

c. AST

d. ALT

148. **Which of the following is the preferred test for hepatic damage in sheep and cattle?**

a. SDH

b. AST

c. ALT

d. None of these

149. **Which of the following is a practical routine test for the evaluation of liver amyloidosis in horses?**

a. GGT

b. BSP

c. Arginase

d. None of these

150. **Serum GGT activity is not valuable in:**

a. Cattle

b. Horses

c. Sheep

d. Dogs

151. **Which of the following tests is preferred for biliary obstruction?**

a. Alkaline phosphatase

b. AST

c. GGT

d. All of these

152. **Which of the following hepatic enzymes is not useful in identifying chromic hepatic disease in cattle?**

a. ALP (alkaline phosphatase)

b. GGT (gamma-glutamyl transferase)

c. GD (glutamate dehydrogenase)

d. ALT (Alamine amino transferase)

153. **The early stages of hepatic dysfunction in cattle can be detected by estimation of:**

a. SDH (sorbitol dehydrogenase)

b. ALP (alkaline phosphatase)

c. Arginase

d. None of these

154. **White liver disease in sheep occurs due to a deficiency of:**

   a. Co

   b. Cu

   c. Fe

   d. None of these

155. **Hepatic failure in horses is caused by:**

   a. Serum hepatitis

   b. Theiler's disease

   c. Acute liver atrophy

   d. All of these

156. **The ruminal and abomasal 'ping' is distinguished using:**

   a. Lip-tik test

   b. BSP – clearance test

   c. Gastroscopy

   d. None of these

157. **LDA is most commonly associated with:**

   a. Prepartum

   b. Postpartum

   c. a and b

   d. None of these

158. **The incidence of LD is higher in which temperatures?**

   a. Cold season

   b. Hot season

   c. Mild season

   d. All of these

159. **Greenish-black ruminal fluid indicates:**

   a. Vagus indigestion

   b. Acid indigestion

c. Simple indigestion

d. All of these

160. **The normal odour of the rumen is:**

a. Aromatic

b. Sour

c. Sweetish

d. None of these

161. **Which of the following is the most reliable test to access the microbial status of the rumen?**

a. MBR

b. Cellulose digestion

c. Glucose termination

d. None of these

162. **Which of the following volatile fatty acids is higher in normal rumen liquor?**

a. Propionic acid

b. Acetic acid

c. Butyric cow

d. None of these

163. **In USG, the gall bladder appears:**

a. Anechoic

b. Hyperechoic

c. Hypoechoic

d. None of these

164. **An L-shaped rumen on rectal examination is found in:**

a. Vagal indigestion

b. Ruminal acidosis

c. Simple indigestion

d. All of these

165. **Paralytic ileus is also known as:**

   a. Adynamic ileus

   b. Dynamic ileus

   c. Mechanical ileus

   d. None of these

166. **Failure of the reticular groove reflex in calves is called:**

   a. Ruminal drinking

   b. Ruminal parakeratosis

   c. Reticular impaction

   d. None of these

167. **Tyzzer disease is most commonly found in:**

   a. Calves

   b. Foals

   c. Dogs

   d. None of these

168. **Lamb dysentery is caused by:**

   a. *Clostridium perfringens* B

   b. *Clostridium perfringens* C

   c. *Clostridium perfringens* A

   d. None of these

169. ***Clostridium perfringens* type C causes:**

   a. Lamb dysentery

   b. Struck

   c. Pulpy kidney disease

   d. All of these

170. **Potomac horse fever is caused by:**

   a. Rickettsia

   b. Bacteria

c. Virus

d. Sheep

171. **Transmissible gastroenteritis is a disease of:**

a. Swine

b. Equines

c. Ruminants

d. Sheep

172. **Swine dysentery is caused by:**

a. Spirochete

b. *Rickettsia*

c. Protozoa

d. None of these

173. **Black, tarry faeces is called:**

a. Dysentery

b. Melena

c. Haematochezia

d. All of these

174. **Stick and tenacious faeces are commonly seen in:**

a. Vagal indigestion

b. Chronic peritonitis

c. Obstruction of the stomach

d. All of these

175. **Spontaneous grunt in cattle is due to:**

a. Diffuse peritonitis

b. Pneumonia

c. Pulmonary emphysema

d. None of these

176. **Absence of faeces for more than 36–48 hours indicates:**

   a. Physical obstruction

   b. Functional obstruction

   c. a and b

   d. None of these

177. **Ruminal hyperkeratosis is caused by:**

   a. Lactic acidosis

   b. Alkaline indigestion

   c. Acetonaemia

   d. None of these

178. **Which of the following have potential to control ruminal acidosis in dairy cattle?**

   a. Monensin

   b. Laidlomycin

   c. Inadequate intake of forage

   d. None of these

179. **Bloat in cattle occurs due to eating:**

   a. Grass pasture with high protein content

   b. Forage containing tannins

   c. Mature plants

   d. None of these

180. **Hoflund syndrome is also known as:**

   a. Acid indigestion

   b. Vagal indigestion

   c. Alkaline indigestion

   d. None of these

181. **Which of the following is a common complication of LDA?**

   a. Ketosis

   b. Acidosis

c. Alkaline indigestion

d. None of these

182. **Most of the rumen gum is eructed in the:**

a. Primary contraction cycle

b. Secondary contraction cycle

c. a and b

d. None of these

183 **Which of the following vitamins is deficient in carbohydrate engorgement in cattle?**

a. B2

b. B6

c. B12

d. B1

184. **A sweet/sour smell of faeces is characteristic of:**

a. Carbohydrate engorgement

b. Alkaline indigestion

c. Protein indigestion

d. None of these

185. **Invagination of one portion of the intestine into the lumen of adjacent segments of the intestine is called:**

a. Intussusception

b. Volvulus

c. Ileus

d. Gut tie

186. **Abomasal bloat in calves can be treated without any adverse effect with:**

a. Formalin 0.1%

b. Formalin 1%

c. Formalin 0.025%

d. None of these

187. **The following condition develops in abomasal impaction:**

    a. Alkalosis with hyperchloremia

    b. Alkalosis with hyporchloremia

    c. Acidosis with hyperchloremia

    d. All of these

188. **The primary cycle contraction of the reticulo rumen involves:**

    a. Biphagic contraction of reticulum

    b. Monophagic contraction of rumen

    c. Polyphagic contraction of rumen

    d. None of these

189. **The presence of a plug of meconium in the rectum indicates:**

    a. Paralytic ileus

    b. Enteritis

    c. Dysentery

    d. All of these

190. **Which of the following tests is used to detect protein-losing enteropathy?**

    a. Starch digestion test

    b. Radioactive isotopes

    c. Glucose

    d. Lactose digestion test

191. **A starch digestion test is used to evaluate:**

    a. Gastric function

    b. Small intestine function

    c. Pancreatic function

    d. All of these

192. **Which of the following animal species have true vomition?**

a. Pigs

b. Cattle

c. Goats

d. Hares

193. **Turbidity of peritoneal fluid indicates:**

a. Increased leucocytes

b. Increased protein

c. Increased fine strands of fibrin

d. All of these

194. **The normal colour of peritoneal fluid in horses is:**

a. Pale yellow

b. Amber

c. Turbid

d. All of these

195. **Which of the following drugs is used to increase gut motility?**

a. Metoclopramide

b. Cisapride

c. a and b

d. None of these

196. **Which of the following is used to treat GI and urinary bladder disorders?**

a. Bethanechol

b. Neostigmine

c. Naloxone

d. All of these

197. **Which of the following may be used in caecal dilatation?**

   a. Bethanechol

   b. Xylazine

   c. Naloxone

   d. None of these

198. **A 'saw horse' stance is suggestive of:**

   a. Diarrhoea

   b. Colic

   c. Dysentery

   d. All of these

199. **In horses, thrombo-embolic colic is caused by:**

   a. Sand

   b. Strongylus vulgaris

   c. Impaction

   d. All of these

200. **Proliferative ileitis occurs in:**

   a. Pigs

   b. Horses

   c. Sheep

   d. None of these

Answers

1.	a	31.	a	61.	a	91.	a
2.	a	32.	a	62.	a	92.	a
3.	a	33.	a	63.	b	93.	a
4.	b	34.	a	64.	a	94.	a
5.	c	35.	a	65.	d	95.	b
6.	d	36.	c	66.	d	96.	a
7.	a	37.	a	67.	a	97.	a
8.	d	38.	a	68.	a	98.	a
9.	d	39.	c	69.	a	99.	b
10.	a	40.	d	70.	b	100.	b
11.	a	41.	d	71.	a	101.	c
12.	a	42.	a	72.	a	102.	a
13.	a	43.	a	73.	a	103.	b
14.	c	44.	a	74.	a	104.	a
15.	d	45.	a	75.	c	105.	a
16.	b	46.	a	76.	a	106.	b
17.	b	47.	b	77.	c	107.	b
18.	a	48.	c	78.	a	108.	d
19.	d	49.	b	79.	d	109.	a
20.	a	50.	a	80.	a	110.	b
21.	a	51.	d	81.	c	111.	d
22.	c	52.	c	82.	c	112.	a
23.	a	53.	a	83.	a	113.	c
24.	c	54.	b	84.	a	114.	a
25.	d	55.	b	85.	a	115.	a
26.	a	56.	d	86.	a	116.	a
27.	b	57.	a	87.	d	117.	a
28.	b	58.	a	88.	d	118.	b
29.	d	59.	d	89.	d	119.	a
30.	c	60.	a	90.	a	120.	a

(Continued)

121.	a	141.	a	161.	a	181.	a
122.	b	142.	d	162.	b	182.	b
123.	d	143.	a	163.	a	183.	d
124.	a	144.	a	164.	a	184.	a
125.	a	145.	c	165.	a	185.	a
126.	a	146.	c	166.	a	186.	a
127.	b	147.	d	167.	b	187.	b
128.	d	148.	a	168.	a	188.	a
129.	a	149.	a	169.	b	189.	a
130.	b	150.	d	170.	a	190.	b
131.	a	151.	a	171.	a	191.	d
132.	a	152.	d	172.	a	192.	a
133.	a	153.	a	173.	b	193.	d
134.	a	154.	a	174.	d	194.	a
135.	c	155.	d	175.	a	195.	c
136.	a	156.	a	176.	c	196.	a
137.	a	157.	b	177.	a	197.	a
138.	b	158.	a	178.	a	198.	b
139.	b	159.	a	179.	a	199.	b
140.	a	160.	a	180.	b	200.	a

9 Diseases of the Liver and Pancreas

Praveen Kumar and Kanchan Arya

Introduction

The liver is the largest parenchymal organ, weighing around 3% of body weight in adults and 5% in young animals. The liver performs numerous functions, including lipid, carbohydrate and protein metabolism; storage, metabolism and activation of vitamins; storage of minerals, glycogen and triglycerides; extramedullary haematopoiesis; synthesis of coagulant and anticoagulant; and detoxification of many endogenous and exogenous compounds, toxins and xenobiotics.

The pancreas has both endocrine and exocrine functions. The exocrine pancreas synthesizes and secretes digestive enzymes (e.g. amylase, lipase, etc.) and inactive proenzymes (trypsinogen, chymotrypsinogen, etc.), which are essential for the digestion of dietary components such as proteins, triglycerides and complex carbohydrates. It also secretes bicarbonate, which buffers gastric acid, an intrinsic factor needed for cobalamin absorption.

Clinical signs of hepatobiliary and pancreatic diseases are variable and non-specific in dogs and cats. Vomiting, diarrhoea and anorexia are common clinical signs associated with both pancreas and liver disease. Jaundice, abdominal pain, polyuria and polydipsia, abdominal effusion, hepatomegaly, coagulopathies, photosensitization, protein calorie malnutrition are also the clinical manifestation of liver and pancreatic diseases. Jaundice or icterus is the yellow staining of unpigmented skin, mucosal and conjunctival membranes, serum or tissues by an excessive amount of bile pigment or bilirubin in blood. Jaundice may be pre-hepatic, due to very marked red cell breakdown; hepatic, due to primary liver disease; or post hepatic, due to biliary tract obstruction or rupture. Neurologic dysfunction was described in patients with liver disease as a result of exposure of the cerebral cortex to toxic substances (ammonia) present in blood that are normally detoxified by the liver. The diagnosis of either liver or pancreatic disease is challenging and relies on a combination of clinicopathologic tests, diagnostic imaging, and often also some form of biopsy, particularly for the liver. Biochemical tests for the hepatobiliary involvement are ALT, AST, ALP, GGT, bilirubin, while to assess function total protein, A:G ratio, bile acid, cholesterol, ammonia, urea, glucose, coagulation tests are performed. Biochemical tests for the pancreatitis are pancreatic lipase immunoreactivity, lipase, amylase, trypsin-like immunoreactivity, cobalamin and blood count, electrolytes, urea and creatinine, etc. In treatment, the main aim should be to remove the source of the damaging agent.

Multiple Choice Questions

1. **What is the shape of the pancreas in dogs?**

   a. Triangular

   b. V

   c. Oval

   d. Human footprint

2. **The degree of pigmentation in icterus is measured by:**

   a. Van Den Bergh test

   b. Cherry Crandall method

   c. Icteric index

   d. Roe-Byler method

3. **The most accurate method for detection of fatty infiltration in the liver of farm animals is:**

   a. Liver biopsy

   b. USG

   c. Biochemical tests

   d. Urine examination

4. **Oral hypoglycaemic drugs include:**

   a. Sulfonylurea

   b. Isophane (NPH)

   c. Lente

   d. Protamine zinc (PZI)

5. **Biphasic van den Bergh's reaction is seen in:**

   a. Pre-hepatic jaundice

   b. Hepatic jaundice

   c. Post-hepatic jaundice

   d. All of these

6. **Serum lipase estimation methods include:**

   a. Cherry Crandall method

   b. Roe-Byler method

   c. a and b

   d. None of these

7. **Necrotic hepatitis is caused by**

   a. *Clostridium haemolyticum*

   b. *Clostridium novyi* type B

   c. *Mycoplasma* spp.

   d. *Aspergillus* spp.

8. **Icteric appearance of the carcass, hepatomegaly and distinctive bronze-coloured liver is seen in:**

   a. Fowl typhoid

   b. Pullorum disease

   c. Fowl cholera

   d. None of these

9. **The blood glucose level in ketosis is:**

   a. 60–70mg/dl

   b. 50–60 mg/dl

   c. 10–20mg/dl

   d. 20–40 mg/dl

10. **Lupinosis, characterized by jaundice and yellow atrophy of the liver, occurs due to:**

    a. Deficiency of methionine

    b. Ingestion of *Lantana camara*

    c. Mycotoxin *Phomopsis*

    d. All of these

11. **Bile acids are formed due to the metabolism of:**

    a. Proteins

    b. Cholesterol

    c. Bile pigments

    d. Amino acids

12. **Gall bladder tumours are quite large in size and are mostly of what type?**

    a. Hemangiosarcoma

    b. Papillary cystadenomas

    c. Lymphosarcoma

    d. Myelosarcoma

13. **Neonatal foals have a higher concentration of which enzyme?**

    a. AST

    b. ALT

    c. SDH

    d. GGT

14. **Metabolite of chlorophyll is commonly implicated in hepatogenous photosensitization, and results in the production of:**

    a. Phylloerythrin

    b. Erythrins

    c. a and b

    d. None of these

15. **In biliary patency and hepatocyte function, structure and blood flow are evaluated by:**

    a. Ultrasonography

    b. Echocardiography

    c. Scintigraphy

    d. Liver biopsy

16. **Which dye is used to access hepatobiliary transport?**

    a. Sulfobromophthalein (BSP) dye

    b. Bromothymol blue dye

    c. Bromocresol purple dye

    d. b and c

17. **Tyzzer disease is characterized by acute necrotizing hepatitis, myocarditis and colitis in foals. What is its cause?**

    a. *Salmonella*

    b. *Clostridium*

    c. *Herpes virus*

    d. *Pseudomonas*

18. **Which fungus causes cholangiohepatitis in sheep and cattle?**

    a. *Aspergillus spp.*

    b. *Pithomyces chartarum*

    c. a and b

    d. None of these

19. **The primary etiological agent of hepatic abscess in cattle is:**

    a. *Corynebacterium*

    b. *Salmonella*

    c. *E. coli*

    d. *Fusobacterium necrophorum*

20. **The etiological agent of hepatic abscess in goats is:**

    a. *Corynebacterium pseudotuberculosis*

    b. *Trueperella pyogenes*

    c. *E. coli*

    d. All of these

21. **White liver disease in sheep is caused by:**

    a. Cobalt deficiency

    b. Vitamin A deficiency

c. Selenium and vitamin E deficiency

d. None of these

22. **Serum hepatitis/postvaccinal hepatitis/Theiler's disease is the most common cause of acute hepatic failure in:**

a. Cattle

b. Dogs

c. Horses

d. Cats

23. **Pre-hepatic jaundice is caused by:**

a. Equine infectious anaemia

b. Babesiosis

c. Chronic copper poisoning

d. All of these

24. **In icterus, yellow pigmentation occurs in which sequence?**

a. Skin, conjunctiva, urine, blood

b. Conjunctiva, skin, blood, urine

c. Blood, urine, conjunctiva, skin

d. Urine, skin, blood, conjunctiva

25. **Which of the following is a common liver disease in cattle?**

a. Fatty liver

b. Hepatitis

c. Cirrhosis

d. Cholangitis

26. **Which of the following vitamins is essential for proper liver function in farm animals?**

a. Vitamin C

b. Vitamin D

c. Vitamin E

d. Vitamin K

27. **Hyperketonaemia and hypoglycaemia are characteristic of:**

   a. Milk fever

   b. Downer cow

   c. Fatty liver syndrome

   d. None of these

28. **Hemochromatosis in cattle is deposition of:**

   a. Hemosiderin

   b. Bile pigment

   c. a and b

   d. None of these

29. **Chronic diffuse hepatitis characterized by progressive or recurrent destruction of liver cell is due to:**

   a. Autoimmune causes

   b. *D. mellitus*

   c. Congestive heart failure

   d. All of these

30. **Hepatic abscesses are a common cause of liver disease in:**

   a. Cattle

   b. Horses, dogs and cats

   c. Pigs and cattle

   d. Sheep and goats

31. **Clinical icterus in ruminants is most frequently associated with:**

   a. Liver disease

   b. Haemolytic crisis

   c. Biliary stasis

   d. None of these

32. **Encephalopathy associated with liver disease is a prominent feature in:**

   a. Horses and cattle

   b. Dogs and cattle

   c. Sheep and goats

   d. All of these

33. **Hepatosis is characterized by:**

   a. Inflammation

   b. Degeneration

   c. Metabolism

   d. b and c

34. **The type of icterus in which the level of conjugate bilirubin greatly increases is known as:**

   a. Post-hepatic

   b. Hepatic

   c. Pre-hepatic

   d. None of these

35. **Conjugate bilirubin in a urine sample can be demonstrated by:**

   a. Diazo tablet test

   b. Gomelin-Rosenbach test

   c. Methylene blue test

   d. All of these

36. **Gradual loss of body condition, poor appetite, debility and constipation are characteristic features of:**

   a. Toxic hepatitis

   b. Pre-hepatic jaundice

   c. Liver cirrhosis

   d. None of these

37. **Liver cirrhosis can be confirmed by:**

    a. Liver function test

    b. Liver biopsy

    c. a and b

    d. None of these

38. **Liver cirrhosis can be treated by:**

    a. 2–4 L of 10% dextrose intravenously once or twice daily

    b. 1–2 L of 20% dextrose intravenously once or twice daily

    c. 2–3 L of 50% dextrose intravenously once or twice daily

    d. None of these

39. **Which aflatoxin (AF) is recognized as the most potent hepatic carcinogen in the world?**

    a. AFB_2

    b. AFB_1

    c. AFG_2

    d. AFG_1

40. **The most commonly recognized species which produces aflatoxins (AFs) is:**

    a. *Aspergillus flavus*

    b. *Aspergillus Parasiticus*

    c. *Aspergillus nomius*

    d. All of these

41. **LD_{50} for AFB_1 in calves is:**

    a. 0.5–1.5 mg/kg

    b. 1–2 mg/kg

    c. 2–3 mg/kg

    d. None of these

42. **In the liver, aflatoxins undergo biotransformation, producing which toxic metabolite?**

    a. AFB_1 8–9-epoxide

    b. AFB_1 3–4 -epoxide

    c. a and b

    d. None of these

43. **Which cytochrome is actively involved in the transformation of AFB_1 into toxic metabolite?**

    a. P425

    b. P456

    c. P450

    d. P230

44. **Fatty liver in large animals most commonly occurs during:**

    a. Immediate post-parturition

    b. First two weeks after parturition

    c. First month after calving

    d. All of these

45. **In cattle, ultrasonographic examination of the liver is performed:**

    a. On the right side of the abdomen from 7th to 12th intercostal space

    b. On the left side of the abdomen from 7th to 12th intercostal space

    c. On the right side of the abdomen from 5th to 4th intercostal space

    d. a and c

46. **Following ultrasonographical examination, grade I (mild) hepatic lipidosis is characterized by:**

    a. Bright pattern with vessel blurring and marked deep attenuation

    b. Bright pattern with vessel blurring, no marked deep attenuation

c. Homogenous granular echo texture with clear and sharp margins

d. a and b

47. **The gold standard test for ketosis in dairy animals is:**

a. Blood β- hydroxy butyrate (BHB)

b. Acetoacetate and acetone in urine

c. Low concentration of blood glucose

d. a and c

48. **Photosensitization is a feature of poisoning with:**

a. Datura

b. Lantana

c. Abrus

d. Bracken fern

49. **Haemoglobinuria, associated with hepatitis, is common in:**

a. Horses

b. Cattle

c. Cats

d. Pigs

50. **Eclampsia in bitches is treated with:**

a. 50% dextrose

b. 10% calcium gluconate

c. a and b

d. Thiamine

51. **Ovine ketosis is characterized by:**

a. High plasma cortisol

b. High plasma glucose

c. High plasma potassium

d. None of these

52. **Hepatosis dietetica in swine is caused by:**

    a. Feeding a high energy diet

    b. Excess of unsaturated fatty acid

    c. Deficiency of vitamin E and Se

    d. All of these

53. **Primary ketosis is also called:**

    a. Production disease

    b. Starvation disease

    c. Ketosis due to nutritional deficiency

    d. Alimentary ketosis

54. **The cyst of *Echinococcus granulosus* is mainly found in the:**

    a. Liver

    b. Lungs

    c. a and b

    d. Kidneys

55. **Which vitamin is indicated in biliary obstruction?**

    a. Vitamin B complex

    b. Vitamin K

    c. Vitamin C

    d. Vitamin A

56. **Hepatic insufficiency in dogs is treated with which type of diet?**

    a. Plenty of glucose

    b. Protein with high biological value

    c. Low fat or fat-free

    d. All of these

57. **Offensive odour, clay coloured, putrid and putty faeces is observed in:**

   a. Hepatic jaundice

   b. Obstructive jaundice

   c. Pre-hepatic jaundice

   d. All of these

58. **The most satisfactory instrument or method for liver biopsy is:**

   a. Tru-cut needle

   b. Trocar canula

   c. Percutaneous biopsy

   d. a and b

59. **What is the normal bilirubin level in pigs?**

   a. 0–0.4 mg/dl

   b. 0–1.9mg/dl

   c. 0–0.2 mg/dl

   d. 1–10 mg/dl

60. **Parasitic hepatitis is caused by:**

   a. Migratory larvae of *Ascaris* spp.

   b. *Fasciola gigantica*

   c. *Fasciloa hepatica*

   d. All of these

61. **Hepatitis due to dietary deficiency is also known as:**

   a. Trophopathic hepatitis

   b. Nutritional hepatitis

   c. Dietary hepatitis

   d. None of these

62. **Dummy syndrome is:**

   a. Hypoglycaemic encephalopathy

   b. Photosensitizing dermatitis

   c. Haemorrhagic diathesis

   d. None of these

63. **Glycogen storage disease in dogs is due to deficiency of which enzyme?**

   a. Glucose-6phosphate

   b. Alkaline phosphate

   c. Ceruloplasmin

   d. Adenylate cyclase

64. **The most common circulatory anomalies of the liver in dogs are:**

   a. Microvascular dysplasia (MDA)

   b. Portosystemic vascular anomalies (PSVAs)

   c. a and b

   d. None of these

65. **A contagious disease of dogs characterized by biphasic fever, congestion of the mucous membrane, severe depression-marked leukopenia and coagulation disorder is known as:**

   a. Infectious canine hepatitis

   b. Canine parvovirus

   c. Canine herpes virus

   d. Leptospirosis

66. **Infectious canine hepatitis is caused by:**

   a. Canine adenovirus 2

   b. Canine adenovirus 1

   c. a and b

   d. Calicivirus

67. **Which of the following causes hepatic necrosis and other systemic changes usually affecting neonatal puppies and is highly fatal:**

   a. Canine parvovirus

   b. Canine herpesvirus

   c. Leptospirosis

   d. Calicivirus

68. **Chronic weight loss, polyphagia, hepatomegaly and increased AST and ALT levels in young Abyssinian and Somali cats is due to:**

   a. *Mycobacterium avium*

   b. *Mycobacterium tuberculosis*

   c. *Mycobacterium leprae*

   d. All of these

69. **Nodular cirrhosis occurs in:**

   a. Old dogs

   b. Old cattle

   c. Kids

   d. Sheep

70. **The normal random blood glucose level in dogs is:**

   a. 80–120mg/dl

   b. 40 mg/dl

   c. 50–100 mg/dl

   d. 60–70mg/dl

71. **The dose of protamine zinc insulin in ketosis is:**

   a. 100–200 IU

   b. 200–300 IU

   c. 300–400 IU

   d. None of these

72. **'Pipe stem liver' is characteristic of:**

    a. Ascariasis

    b. Amphistomiasis

    c. Fascioliasis

    d. Schistosomiasis

73. **The 'organ par excellence' is:**

    a. Kidneys

    b. Spleen

    c. Liver

    d. Heart

74. **Trophopathic hepatitis is due to deficiency of:**

    a. Vitamin E

    b. Methionine

    c. a and b

    d. Vitamin A

75. **Yellow tar weed seed (*Amsinka intermedia*) is the toxic cause of which disease?**

    a. Hepatitis

    b. Liver cirrhosis

    c. Jaundice

    d. Peritonitis

76. **Viral disease in horses leads to:**

    a. Equine infectious anaemia (EIA)

    b. Glanders

    c. Strangles

    d. Equine herpesvirus

77. **Toxic hepatitis is due to:**

    a. As

    b. SO, CCl_4

    c. C_2, Cl_2

    d. All of these

78. **In equines, which protozoa causes biliary jaundice?**

    a. Babesia

    b. Theileria

    c. Eimeria

    d. None of these

79. **Which of the following species is more affected with hydatid cyst infection:**

    a. Sheep and buffalo

    b. Goats and pigs

    c. Dogs and cats

    d. Horses and cattle

80. **Which test is used for bile salts in urine?**

    a. Benzidine test

    b. Hay sulphur test

    c. Ascoli test

    d. Alizurine test

81. **Which fungi can be responsible for liver damage?**

    a. Aspergillus

    b. Fusarium

    c. a and b

    d. None of these

82. **Inflammation of the biliary duct system is called:**

    a. Cholangitis

    b. Cholelithiasis

c. Cholecystitis

d. None of these

83. **In fasciolosis, fibrosis of the liver and bile duct is due to release of what, which stimulates collagen production?**

a. Proline

b. Choline

c. Heparin

d. Hyaluronidase enzyme

84. **In canine 'paintbrush', haemorrhages on the gastric serosa, lymph nodes, thymus and pancreas are pathognomic lesions in:**

a. ICH

b. Canine parvovirus

c. Jaundice

d. None of these

85. **How is fowl typhoid treated?**

a. 0.1–0.2% sulphathiazole

b. 0.01–0.1 sulphathiazole

c. a and b

d. 0.5–0.6% sulphathiazole

86. **Defused hepatitis, fatty changes, focal necrosis and diffused infiltration of lymphocytes in the liver are general features of:**

a. Fowl cholera

b. Fowl typhoid

c. Avian paratyphoid

d. None of these

87. **The MAT is widely utilized for the diagnosis of Leptospira. What ratio of titre indicates present or past infection?**

a. 1:1000

b. 1:100

c. 1:200

d. 1:10

88. **The correct dosage for treatment of echinococcosis in canines is:**

a. Fenbendazole (50 mg/kg BWT)

b. Albendazole (12mg/kg BWT)

c. Praziquantel (10mg/kg BWT)

d. Tetramisole (15mg/kg BWT)

89. **In chronic fasciolosis there may be a secondary infection of:**

a. *Clostridium perfringens*

b. *Clostridium botulinum*

c. *Clostridium novyi*

d. None of these

90. **Pregnancy toxaemia in cows is known as:**

a. Whole milk tetany

b. Fatty cow syndrome

c. Grass tetany

d. Downer cow syndrome

91. **Which of these is a risk factor for fatty cow syndrome?**

a. Well-fed and highly obsessed cows

b. High milk yielder

c. a and b

d. Excessive exercise

92. **The most reliable biochemical tests for liver diseases in bovines consist of:**

a. ALT, AST, alkaline phosphatase

b. Glutamate dehydrogenase, ALT

   c. Glutamate dehydrogenase, sorbitol dehydrohenase and gamma glutamyl transferase

   d. Arginase, ALT

93. Hepatitis cysticercosa is caused by:

   a. *Cysticercus cellulosae*

   b. *C. bovis*

   c. Coenurus

   d. *C. tenuicollis*

94. Which is not a test of the liver?

   a. Takata-ara test

   b. Liver biopsy

   c. Prothrombin time

   d. Nitrite reduction test

95. Faecal muscle fibre is known as:

   a. Steatorrhoea

   b. Amylorrhoea

   c. Creatorrhoea

   d. None of these

96. Hepatic encephalopathy is associated with:

   a. High ammonia

   b. High CO_2

   c. High CH_4

   d. High Cl_2

97. Management of hepatic encephalopathy does not include:

   a. Lactulose

   b. Oral probiotic yogurt

   c. Excessive protein restriction

   d. Amoxicillin

98. **Cholelithotripsy is:**

    a. A process of crushing of gall stones

    b. A process of removing bile

    c. A process of removing the gall bladder

    d. None of these

99. **Total serum cholesterol is increased in:**

    a. Hepatic jaundice

    b. Pre-hepatic jaundice

    c. Post-hepatic jaundice

    d. a and c

100. **A pathognomonic sign of pancreatitis in dogs is:**

    a. Cranial abdominal pain

    b. Severe vomiting

    c. Acholic faeces

    d. None of these

101. **Which is a negative prognostic indicator of pancreatitis?**

    a. Acute pancreatitis

    b. Chronic pancreatitis

    c. More severe clinical signs

    d. a and c

102. **Pre-hepatic jaundice is characterized by:**

    a. Absence of bilirubin in the urine

    b. Clay-coloured faeces

    c. Increase in urobilinogen in the urine

    d. a and c

103. **Urobilinogen is absent in urine of animals suffering from:**

   a. Pre-hepatic jaundice

   b. Post-hepatic jaundice

   c. Hepatic jaundice

   d. All of these

104. **Acholic faeces is characteristic of**

   a. Haemolytic Jaundice

   b. Hepatocellular jaundice

   c. Cholestatic jaundice

   d. Overproduction jaundice

105. **The most common cause of jaundice in cattle is:**

   a. Haemolytic diseases

   b. Degeneration of liver cells

   c. Obstruction of bile duct

   d. Hepatitis

106. **Which of these is a negative prognostic indicator in dogs with chronic hepatitis?**

   a. Ascites

   b. Jaundice

   c. a and b

   d. None of these

107. **The most common disorder associated with exocrine pancreas is:**

   a. Exocrine pancreatic insufficiency

   b. Pancreatitis

   c. Pancreatic adenocarcinoma

   d. Pancreatic abscess

108. **Abdominal pain is present in:**

   a. Hepatomegaly

   b. Acute pancreatitis

   c. EBDO

   d. All of these

109. **The classical sign of a 'praying stance' in dogs is seen due to pain in the:**

   a. Liver

   b. Pancreas

   c. Stomach or duodenum

   d. All of these

110. **Chronic exocrine pancreatic insufficiency will not be apparent until how much acinar tissue is lost (approximately)?**

   a. 75%

   b. 100%

   c. 90%

   d. 50%

111. **Pancreatic acinar cells secrete:**

   a. Amylase and lipase

   b. Bicarbonate

   c. Intrinsic factor

   d. All of these

112. **The diagnostic test for exocrine pancreatic insufficiency in dogs is:**

   a. Trypsin-like immunoreactivity (TLI)

   b. Pancreatic lipase immunoreactivity (PLI)

   c. Serum amylase activity

   d. Faecal elastase

113. **The most specific diagnostic test for pancreatitis is:**

    a. PLI

    b. TLI

    c. Contrast-enhanced ultrasonography

    d. Pancreatic biopsy

114. **Acute pancreatitis results in a decreased concentration of what in the serum of dogs?**

    a. Urea

    b. Potassium

    c. GGT

    d. ALT

115. **Acute pancreatitis results in an increased concentration of what in the blood of dogs?**

    a. Potassium

    b. Urea and creatinine

    c. Chloride

    d. Platelets

116. **In dogs, steatorrhea with yellow, smelly, voluminous faeces is associated with disease of the:**

    a. Liver

    b. Gall bladder

    c. Pancreas

    d. Intestine

117. **The presence of glucose and ketones in the urine of a dog with pancreatitis usually indicates:**

    a. Ketosis

    b. Diabetes mellitus

    c. Diabetic ketoacidosis

    d. EPI

118. **The gold standard test for diagnosis of pancreatitis is:**

    a. Biopsy

    b. TLI

    c. USG

    d. Serum lipaseactivity

119. **A risk factor for pancreatitis in dogs is:**

    a. Potassium bromide

    b. High fat diet

    c. Surgery

    d. All of these

120. **The most effective antiemetic used in dogs with acute pancreatitis is:**

    a. Metoclopromide

    b. Phenothiazine

    c. Maropitant

    d. All of these

121. **Which drug should be avoided in dogs with pancreatitis?**

    a. Antiemetic

    b. NSAID

    c. Gastroprotectant

    d. Fluid therapy

122. **The most common clinical finding in pancreatitis is:**

    a. Vomition

    b. Abdominal pain

    c. Anorexia and weakness

    d. All of these

123. **Abdominal pain in pancreatitis is treated with:**

   a. NSAID

   b. Morphine

   c. Fentanyl

   d. b and c

124. **Exocrine pancreatic insufficiency (EPI) is mainly caused by:**

   a. Inflammation of the pancreas

   b. Decreased production of digestive enzymes

   c. Tumour of the pancreas

   d. Hyperacidity of the duodenum

125. **Treatment of dogs and cats with EPI includes supplementation with:**

   a. Digestive enzymes

   b. Cobalamin

   c. a and b

   d. None of these

126. **Diagnosis of exocrine pancreatic insufficiency (EPI) is performed by:**

   a. Pancreatic function tests

   b. Biopsy

   c. Clinical signs

   d. a and c

127. **Which vitamin is deficient in dogs affected by EPI?**

   a. B12

   b. A

   c. C

   d. B1

128. **Which of the following is false for exocrine pancreatic insufficiency?**

   a. TLI is decreased

   b. Pancreatic enzymes should be measured after feeding

   c. It is not necessary to stop exogenous pancreatic enzyme supplementation before measuring TLI

   d. A fat-restricted diet should be given

129. **The prognosis for dogs with pancreatic adenocarcinoma is:**

   a. Grave

   b. Poor

   c. Good

   d. Excellent

130. **Which of these is an endocrine disorder of the pancreas?**

   a. EPI

   b. Pancreatitis

   c. Pancreatic adenomas

   d. Diabetes mellitus

131. **Diabetes mellitus is a disorder of which metabolism?**

   a. Fat

   b. Protein

   c. Carbohydrate

   d. All of these

132. **Diabetes mellitus can be diagnosed by the presence of:**

   a. Persistent hyperglycaemia

   b. Glycosuria

   c. Elevated serum fructosamine

   d. All of these

133. **The initial insulin of choice in cats diagnosed with diabetes mellitus should be:**

   a. Short acting

   b. Long acting

   c. Intermediate acting

   d. Ultra-short acting

134. **The type of insulin given in diabetic ketoacidosis is:**

   a. Regular crystalline insulin

   b. Neutral protamine hagedorn

   c. Protamine zinc insulin

   d. Insulin glargine

135. **Complications of diabetes mellitus include:**

   a. Cataracts and recurring infections

   b. Plantigrade posture in cats

   c. Ketoacidosis

   d. All of these

136. **Which of the following drugs is used to control hypergly-caemia?**

   a. Acarbose

   b. Glipizide

   c. Insulin

   d. All of these

137. **Treatment of IDDM includes:**

   a. Oral sulfonylurea drugs

   b. Diet and weight loss

   c. Insulin

   d. b and c

138. **For treatment of emaciated diabetic dogs, the diet should have:**

    a. High fibre

    b. High simple sugars

    c. Low fibre

    d. Low fat

139. **Portal hypertension is caused by:**

    a. Pre-hepatic causes

    b. Hepatic causes

    c. Post-hepatic causes

    d. All of these

140. **Which gallstone is associated with bacterial infection and biliary stasis?**

    a. Brown pigment stones

    b. Black pigment stones

    c. a and b

    d. None of these

141. **Which of the following is a function of the liver in animals?**

    a. Activation of vitamins

    b. Detoxification

    c. Extramedullary haematopoiesis

    d. All of these

Answers

1.	b	31.	b	61.	a	91.	c
2.	c	32.	c	62.	a	92.	c
3.	a	33.	d	63.	a	93.	d
4.	a	34.	a	64.	c	94.	d
5.	b	35.	d	65.	a	95.	c
6.	c	36.	c	66.	b	96.	a
7.	b	37.	b	67.	b	97.	c
8.	a	38.	a	68.	a	98.	a
9.	d	39.	b	69.	a	99.	c
10.	c	40.	d	70.	a	100.	d
11.	b	41.	a	71.	a	101.	d
12.	b	42.	a	72.	c	102.	d
13.	d	43.	c	73.	c	103.	b
14.	a	44.	d	74.	c	104.	c
15.	c	45.	a	75.	b	105.	a
16.	a	46.	b	76.	a	106.	c
17.	b	47.	a	77.	d	107.	b
18.	b	48.	b	78.	a	108.	d
19.	d	49.	a	79.	b	109.	d
20.	d	50.	b	80.	b	110.	c
21.	a	51.	a	81.	c	111.	d
22.	c	52.	c	82.	a	112.	a
23.	d	53.	a	83.	a	113.	a
24.	c	54.	c	84.	a	114.	b
25.	a	55.	b	85.	a	115.	b
26.	c	56.	d	86.	b	116.	c
27.	c	57.	b	87.	b	117.	c
28.	a	58.	a	88.	c	118.	a
29.	d	59.	c	89.	c	119.	d
30.	a	60.	d	90.	b	120.	c

(Continued)

121.	b	127.	a	133.	b	139.	d
122.	d	128.	b	134.	a	140.	a
123.	d	129.	a	135.	d	141.	d
124.	b	130.	d	136.	d		
125.	c	131.	c	137.	d		
126.	d	132.	d	138.	c		

10 Diseases of the Musculoskeletal System

Shashi Pradhan, Aditya Pratap, Ranbir S. Jatav and Akansha Singh

Introduction

Muscles, ligaments, tendons, cartilage and bones make up the musculoskeletal system. The system's main purposes are to support the body, provide motion and safeguard essential organs. Important hematopoietic system components are found in the skeletal system, which also functions as the body's primary calcium and phosphorus storage system. The neurological, circulatory and integumentary systems, among many others, are interconnected, and illnesses in any one of them can have an impact on the musculoskeletal system as well as complicate diagnosis.

Lameness is typically caused by musculoskeletal diseases. Lameness is an irregular stance or gait brought on by discomfort, mechanical limitations like the patella of horses being fixed upward, or neuromuscular diseases. Pain is the most frequent factor in lameness in all animals. The nature and seriousness of the issue determine the degree of impairment. Lameness is most frequently caused by skeletal, articular and tendon/ligament problems.

Musculoskeletal injuries are a major cause of crippling pain, financial loss and loss of athleticism in horses and dogs. In middle-aged and older animals, osteoarthritis is frequent and has a significant financial impact on horse owners. Acute traumatic injuries are the most frequent cause of musculoskeletal dysfunction in young performance horses. Another typical disabling condition in horses used for performance is a tendon or ligament injury. Cranial cruciate ligament injury causes lameness in dogs, with subsequent osteoarthritis.

© CAB International 2024. *Key Questions in Clinical Farm Animal Medicine Volume 1: Principles of Disease Examination, Diagnosis and Management* (ed. T. Rana) DOI: 10.1079/9781800624788.0010

Although perhaps less frequent, the musculoskeletal system can be negatively impacted by primary muscular diseases, neurologic deficits, toxins, endocrine aberrations, metabolic disorders, infectious diseases, blood and vascular disorders, nutritional imbalances or deficits and, occasionally, congenital defects.

Multiple Choice Questions

1. **The locomotor system is important in maintaining what in animals?**

   a. Posture

   b. Gait

   c. a and b

   d. None of these

2. **Examination of the locomotor organs is what type of examination?**

   a. Physical

   b. Orthopaedic

   c. Clinical

   d. None of these

3. **What produces unstable bone matrix?**

   a. Fluoride deficiency

   b. Excess fluoride

   c. a and b

   d. None of these

4. **Which type of diet inhibits osteoblastic activity?**

   a. Excess copper

   b. Deficient copper

   c. Copper rich

   d. None of these

5. **Low calcium combined with what brings about poor bone growth?**

   a. High magnesium

   b. Low magnesium

   c. a and b

   d. None of these

6. **What produces muscle incoordination and poor bone development?**

   a. High magnesium

   b. Low magnesium

   c. a and b

   d. None of these

7. **What causes alteration in the diaphysis of the bone?**

   a. Excess lead

   b. Lead deficiency

   c. a and b

   d. None of these

8. **What brings about poor osteoblastic activity and resultant osteopenia?**

   a. Low zinc levels

   b. High zinc levels

   c. Normal zinc levels

   d. None of these

9. **Low activity of which vitamin impairs osteoblastic activity?**

   a. A

   b. C

   c. D

   d. K

10. **Low levels of which vitamin may bring about rickets?**

   a. A

   b. C

   c. D

   d. K

11.   **Grade III lameness is considered as being:**

   a. Mild

   b. Moderate

   c. Pronounced

   d. Severe

12.   **Gait is to be observed while the animal is:**

   a. Sitting

   b. Walking

   c. Playing

   d. All of these

13.   **Which grade of lameness is almost undetectable?**

   a. I

   b. II

   c. III

   d. IV

14.   **_____ causes synovial fluid to be viscous.**

   a. Hydrochloric acid

   b. Hyaluronic acid

   c. Acetic acid

   d. Boric acid

15.   **The protein content of synovial fluid is less than:**

   a. 1 g/100ml

   b. 2 g/100ml

   c. 3 g/100ml

   d. 4 g/100ml

16.   **What is the cell count of synovial fluid per mm³?**

   a. 150

   b. 200

c. 250

d. 300

17. _____ are absent in synovial fluid.

    a. RBC

    b. WBC

    c. a and b

    d. None of these

18. Osteomalacia is also known as:

    a. Rickets

    b. Adult rickets

    c. Juvenile rickets

    d. None of these

19. Osteomalacia is due to inadequate blood levels of:

    a. Vitamin D3

    b. Phosphorus

    c. a and b

    d. None of these

20. _____ nephritis may be attributable to osteomalacia.

    a. Chronic

    b. Acute

    c. Sub-acute

    d. None of these

21. Rickets is a disease of which age group of animals?

    a. Young

    b. Adult

    c. Old

    d. All of these

22. **Rickets is related to metabolic disturbances of:**

    a. Calcium

    b. Phosphorus

    c. Vitamin D

    d. All of these

23. **Bow leg is found in rickets due to abnormal curvature of ___ bones.**

    a. Long

    b. Flat

    c. Short

    d. None of these

24. **In rickets, condition X-ray film shows what level of density compared to normal bone?**

    a. High level of density

    b. Low level of density

    c. Both

    d. Normal

25. **The daily requirement of vitamin D in cattle is:**

    a. 100 IU

    b. 700 IU

    c. 1500 IU

    d. 3000 IU

26. **The daily requirement of vitamin D in dogs is:**

    a. 100 IU

    b. 700 IU

    c. 1500 IU

    d. 3000 IU

27. **Osteodystrophia fibrosa is also known as:**

    a. Rickets

    b. Adult rickets

    c. Renal rickets

    d. All of these

28. **'Rubber jaw' is a synonym for:**

    a. Rickets

    b. Adult rickets

    c. Renal rickets

    d. All of these

29. **Osteodystrophia fibrosa is a disease of which age of animal?**

    a. Young

    b. Adult

    c. Old

    d. None of these

30. **Osteodystrophia fibros in horses is also known as:**

    a. Big head

    b. Miller's disease

    c. Bran disease

    d. All of these

31. **Renal rickets is related to:**

    a. Hypoparathyroidism

    b. Hyperparathyroidism

    c. a and b

    d. None of these

32. **Non-inflammatory degeneration of _____ muscle is known as myopathy.**

    a. Skeletal

    b. False

c. a and b

d. None of these

33. **Inflammation of the muscle fibres is known as:**

a. Myopathy

b. Myositis

c. Myoencephalitis

d. None of these

34. **The condition in which the bones undergo a process of condensation is called:**

a. Osteopenia

b. Osteopetrosis

c. Epiphysial dysplasia

d. Osteosclerosis

35. **Which of the following bone disorders is hereditary?**

a. Osteopenia

b. Osteopetrosis

c. Epiphysial dysplasia

d. Osteosclerosis

36. **What indicates a reduced amount of bony tissue on the skeleton?**

a. Osteopenia

b. Osteopetrosis

c. Epiphysial dysplasia

d. Osteosclerosis

37. **What indicates a hardening of bony spaces?**

a. Osteopenia

b. Osteopetrosis

c. Epiphysial dysplasia

d. Osteosclerosis

38.   Which condition is also known as Paget's disease?

a. Suppurative osteitis

b. Non-suppurative osteitis

c. Osteitis deformans

d. None of these

39.   Which of these is a chronic disease of the skeleton where there is softening of the bone followed by thickening of the cortex?

a. Suppurative osteitis

b. Non-suppurative osteitis

c. Osteitis deformans

d. None of these

40.   What denotes osteitis resulting from infection?

a. Suppurative osteitis

b. Non-suppurative osteitis

c. Osteitis deformans

d. None of these

41.   Chronic inflammatory conditions of the bone associated with sclerosis and thickening are known as:

a. Suppurative osteitis

b. Non-suppurative osteitis

c. Osteitis deformans

d. None of these

42.   Inflammation of bone due to infection or injury is known as:

a. Osteolysis

b. Osteitis

c. Osteomyelitis

d. None of these

43. **What denotes inflammation of interior bone affecting the marrow space?**

    a. Osteolysis

    b. Osteitis

    c. Osteomyelitis

    d. None of these

44. **What denotes rarefaction of bone?**

    a. Osteolysis

    b. Osteitis

    c. Osteomyelitis

    d. Osteoporosis

45. **Osteoporosis may result from stimulation of which gland?**

    a. Thyroid

    b. Parathyroid

    c. a and b

    d. None of these

46. **When osteoporosis develops in old age, it is known as what?**

    a. Senile osteoporosis

    b. Juvenile osteoporosis

    c. Neurogenic osteoporosis

    d. None of these

47. **Osteopenia is caused by a deficiency of what?**

    a. Vitamin D3

    b. Amino acids

    c. Calcium and phosphorus

    d. All of these

48. **In which condition is there normal production of osteoid tissues and mineralization, but a decrease or cessation of resorption?**

a. Osteolysis

b. Osteitis

c. Osteomyelitis

d. Osteoporosis

49. **Defects in immobilization of osteoclast cells are seen in:**

a. Osteolysis

b. Osteitis

c. Osteopenia

d. Osteoporosis

50. **Which of the following conditions occurs due to a genetic defect?**

a. Osteopenia

b. Osteopetrosis

c. Epiphysial dysplasia

d. Osteosclerosis

51. **In what type of fracture is the cortical end of the fracture forced or impacted into the cancellous bone?**

a. Impacted

b. Compression

c. Avulsion

d. Overriding

52. **In what type of fracture does cancellous bone collapse and compress upon itself?**

a. Impacted

b. Compression

c. Avulsion

d. Overriding

53. **In what type of fracture is a fragment of bone at the insertion point of a tendon or ligament fractured and distracted from the rest of the bone?**

    a. Impacted

    b. Compression

    c. Avulsion

    d. Overriding

54. **In what type of fracture do the fragments lie side by side, causing shortening of the limb?**

    a. Impacted

    b. Compression

    c. Avulsion

    d. Overriding

55. **In what type of fracture are the fragments depressed, producing a cavity?**

    a. Impacted

    b. Compressed

    c. Depression

    d. Distracted

56. **In what type of fracture does the fracture line run transverse to the long axis of the bone?**

    a Transverse

    b. Oblique

    c. a and b

    d. None of these

57. **In what type of fracture does the fracture line run oblique to the long axis of the bone?**

    a. Transverse

    b. Oblique

    c. Spiral

    d. Longitudinal

58. **In what type of fracture does the fracture line spiral along the long axis of the bone?**

    a. Transverse

    b. Oblique

    c. Spiral

    d. Longitudinal

59. **In what type of fracture does the fracture line extend in a longitudinal direction?**

    a. Transverse

    b. Oblique

    c. Spiral

    d. Longitudinal

60. **In what type of fracture is the bone broken into three or more segments?**

    a. Longitudinal

    b. Multiple

    c. Spiral

    d. Oblique

61. **In which type of Salter Harris fracture is the epiphysis displaced from the metaphysis at the growth plate?**

    a. I

    b. II

    c. III

    d. IV

62. **In which type of Salter Harris fracture is a small piece of metaphyseal bone, along with epiphysis, separated from the metaphysis at the growth plate?**

    a. I

    b. II

    c. III

    d. IV

63. In which type of Salter Harris fracture is a small piece of epiphysis and a part of the growth plate fractured, but the metaphysis is unaffected?

   a. I

   b. II

   c. III

   d. IV

64. In which type of Salter Harris fracture is the fracture through the epiphysis, growth plate and metaphysis?

   a. I

   b. II

   c. III

   d. IV

65. In which type of Salter Harris fracture is impaction of the epiphyseal plate, along with the metaphysis, driven into the epiphysis?

   a. I

   b. V

   c. III

   d. II

66. What is defined as a joint injury in which the fibres of supporting ligaments of the joint are ruptured by direct or indirect trauma?

   a. Sprain

   b. Strain

   c. Bursitis

   d. None of these

67. **What is defined as an injury to a muscle or tendon due to overstretching or overuse of any part of the muscle tendon unit?**

    a. Sprain

    b. Strain

    c. Bursitis

    d. None of these

68. **Backward deviation of the carpal joints is known as:**

    a. Calf knee

    b. Goat knee

    c. Knock knee

    d. Bow legs

69. **Forward deviation of the carpal joints is known as:**

    a. Calf knee

    b. Goat knee

    c. Knock knee

    d. Bow legs

70. **Medial deviation of the carpal joints is known as:**

    a. Calf knee

    b. Goat knee

    c. Knock knee

    d. Bow legs

71. **Lateral deviation of the carpal joints is known as:**

    a. Calf knee

    b. Goat knee

    c. Knock knee

    d. Bow legs

72.   **Dorsal deviation of the carpal joints is also known as:**

a. Bucked knee

b. Knee sprung

c. Goat knee

d. All of these

73.   **Medial deviation of the carpal joints is also known as:**

a. Knock knee

b. Carpus valgus

c. Knee narrow

d. All of these

74.   **Irregular profile of the carpal joints which gives the impression that the joints are not fully closed is known as:**

a. Knock knee

b. Open knee

c. Knee narrow

d. Bench knee

75.   **What is the name of the condition in which the metatarsal bone is offset or shifted to the lateral side?**

a. Knock knee

b. Open knee

c. Bench knee

d. Knee narrow

76.   **Inflammation of one or more bones located on the inside of the hock joint is called:**

a. Bone spavin

b. Bog spavin

c. Splints

d. None of these

77. **Soft, spongy bursal enlargement of the hock joint capsule is called:**

    a. Bone spavin

    b. Bog spavin

    c. Splints

    d. None of these

78. **Inflammation of the sheath encasing the tendon from the knee to the fetlock is known as:**

    a. Bowed tendons

    b. Bog spavin

    c. Bone spavin

    d. Capped knee

79. **Bursal enlargement up to the size of a tennis ball on the point of the hock is called:**

    a. Bowed tendons

    b. Capped hocks

    c. Capped knee

    d. Bog spavin

80. **Inflammation on the upper rear of the cannon area just below the point of the hock is referred to as:**

    a. Curb

    b. Jack spavin

    c. Splints

    d. Bog spavin

81. **Bony growth at the back of the knee on inner side is called:**

    a. Curb

    b. Jack spavin

    c. Knee spavin

    d. Bog spavin

82. **Inflammation of the joint capsule in the front of the fetlock joint is called:**

    a. Green osselets

    b. Sesamoditis

    c. Speedy cut

    d. Splint

83. **Bony growth at the front of the fetlock joint is referred to as:**

    a. Osselets

    b. Sesamoditis

    c. Speedy cut

    d. Splint

84. **Inflammation of the bone above and at the back of the fetlock joint is called:**

    a. Green osselets

    b. Sesamoditis

    c. Speedy cut

    d. Splint

85. **Injury due to striking the inner and lower side of the knee with the inside toe of the opposite hoof is known as:**

    a. Green osselets

    b. Sesamoditis

    c. Speedy cut

    d. Splint

86. **Bony enlargements on the insides of the front legs just below the knee are called:**

    a. Green osselets

    b. Sesamoditis

    c. Speedy cut

    d. Splint

87. **Inflammation of the skin that covers the shin bone is known as:**

   a. Shin splints

   b. Sesamoditis

   c. Speedy cut

   d. Splint

88. **Bursal enlargement of the deep digital flexor tendon sheath is referred to as:**

   a. Thoroughpin

   b. Windpuff

   c. Stocking up

   d. Exostosis

89. **Fluid retention in the lower limbs is known as:**

   a. Thoroughpin

   b. Windpuff

   c. Stocking up

   d. Exostosis

90. **Soft, spongy swellings around the back, front and/or side of the fetlock joint are called:**

   a. Thoroughpin

   b. Windpuff

   c. Stocking up

   d. Exostosis

91. **A spur or bony outgrowth from a bone is called a what?**

   a. Thoroughpin

   b. Windpuff

   c. Stocking up

   d. Exostosis

92. **Fixation of a joint due to fusion of the bones is referred to as:**

   a. Thoroughpin

   b. Ankylosis

   c. Stocking up

   d. Exostosis

93. **Renal rickets is related to:**

   a. Hypoparathyroidism

   b. Hyperparathyroidism

   c. a and b

   d. None of these

94. **_____degeneration of skeletal muscle is known as myopathy.**

   a. Non-inflammatory

   b. Inflammatory

   c. Adaptive

   d. None of these

95. **Inflammation of muscle fibres is known as:**

   a. Myopathy

   b. Myositis

   c. Myoencephalitis

   d. None of these

96. **What is the name of the condition in which the bones undergo a process of condensation?**

   a. Osteopenia

   b. Osteopetrosis

   c. Epiphyseal dysplasia

   d. Osteosclerosis

97. Which of the following bone disorders is hereditary?

a. Osteopenia

b. Osteopetrosis

c. Epiphyseal dysplasia

d. Osteosclerosis

98. What causes a reduced amount of bony tissue on the skeleton?

a. Osteopenia

b. Osteopetrosis

c. Epiphyseal dysplasia

d. Osteosclerosis

99. What causes hardening of bony spaces?

a. Osteopenia

b. Osteopetrosis

c. Epiphyseal dysplasia

d. Osteosclerosis

100. Which condition is also known as Paget's disease?

a. Suppurative osteitis

b. Non-suppurative osteitis

c. Osteitis deformans

d. None of these

101. Which of these is a chronic disease of the skeleton where there is softening of the bone followed by thickening of the cortex?

a. Suppurative osteitis

b. Non-suppurative osteitis

c. Osteitis deformans

d. None of these

102. **Which term denotes osteitis resulting from infection?**

   a. Suppurative osteitis

   b. Non-suppurative osteitis

   c. Osteitis deformans

   d. None of these

103. **Which of these diseases affects the vertebrae?**

   a. Ankylosis

   b. Spondylosis

   c. Arthropathy

   d. Dysplasia

104. **Which of these is a disease of the joints?**

   a. Ankylosis

   b. Spondylosis

   c. Arthropathy

   d. Dysplasia

105. **Which of these is a disease process involving the bone growth centres?**

   a. Osteochondrosis

   b. Osteochondritis

   c. Crepitation

   d. Arthrogryposis

106. **Which of these is an inflammatory process involving the bone growth centres?**

   a. Osteochondrosis

   b. Osteochondritis

   c. Crepitation

   d. Arthrogryposis

107. **Which of these creates a creaking, cracking and grating sound?**

   a. Osteochondrosis

   b. Osteochondritis

   c. Crepitation

   d. Arthrogryposis

108. **Permanent contracture of the multiple joints is known as:**

   a. Osteochondrosis

   b. Osteochondritis

   c. Crepitation

   d. Arthrogryposis

109. **Lateral deviation of the vertebral column is called:**

   a. Scoliosis

   b. Kyphosis

   c. Lordosis

   d. Hemiplegia

110. **Dorsal deviation of the vertebral column is called:**

   a. Scoliosis

   b. Kyphosis

   c. Lordosis

   d. Hemiplegia

111. **Ventral deviation of the vertebral column is called:**

   a. Scoliosis

   b. Kyphosis

   c. Lordosis

   d. Hemiplegia

112. **Paralysis of one side of the body is known as:**

    a. Scoliosis

    b. Kyphosis

    c. Lordosis

    d. Hemiplegia

113. **Suprascapular nerve injury resulting in atrophy of the supraspinatus and infraspinatus muscle is known as:**

    a. Sweeny

    b. Bicipital bursitis

    c. Omarthritis

    d. Capped elbow

114. **What is the name for inflammation of intertubercular bursa?**

    a. Sweeny

    b. Bicipital bursitis

    c. Omarthritis

    d. Capped elbow

115. **Arthritis of the scapulohumeral joint is referred to as:**

    a. Sweeny

    b. Bicipital bursitis

    c. Omarthritis

    d. Capped elbow

116. **Appreciable, freely movable swelling over the point of the elbow is referred to as:**

    a. Sweeny

    b. Bicipital bursitis

    c. Omarthritis

    d. Capped elbow

117. **The appearance of dropped elbow is seen in:**

    a. Paralysis of the radial nerve

    b. Bicipital bursitis

    c. Omarthritis

    d. Capped elbow

118. **Acute or chronic inflammation of the carpal joint involving the synovial membrane is seen in:**

    a. Carpitis

    b. Bicipital bursitis

    c. Omarthritis

    d. Radial nerve paralysis

119. **Swelling over the dorsal surface of the carpus, which may be lined by the cells that in turn secrete a fluid is seen in:**

    a. Paralysis of radial nerve

    b. Bicipital bursitis

    c. Hygroma

    d. Capped elbow

120. **A superficial or deep wound on the front of the knees is called:**

    a. Paralysis of the radial nerve

    b. Broken knee

    c. Omarthritis

    d. Capped elbow

121. **A spur or bony outgrowth from a bone is known as a:**

    a. Thoroughpin

    b. Windpuff

    c. Stocking up

    d. Exostosis

122. **What is the correct term for fixation of a joint due to fusion of the bones?**

   a. Thoroughpin

   b. Ankylosis

   c. Stocking up

   d. Exostosis

123. **Renal rickets is related to:**

   a. Hypoparathyroidism

   b. Hyperparathyroidism

   c. a and b

   d. None of these

124. **Non-inflammatory degeneration of the skeletal muscle is known as_____**

   a. Myopathy

   b. Myositis

   c. a and b

   d. None of these

125. **Inflammation of muscle fibres known as:**

   a. Myopathy

   b. Myositis

   c. Myoencephalitis

   d. None of these

126. **A knee wound that heals by superficial intension, leading to a large scar is known as what?**

   a. Blemish knee

   b. Open knee

   c. Hygroma

   d. Contracted tendon

127. **What is commonly acquired in nature and causes pseudo-arthritis resulting from trauma?**

   a. Blemish knee

   b. Open knee

   c. Hygroma

   d. Contracted tendon

128. **An open knee joint also known as:**

   a. Blemish knee

   b. Traumatic arthritis

   c. Hygroma

   d. Contracted tendon

129. **Which of these is a congenital problem?**

   a. Blemish knee

   b. Open knee

   c. Hygroma

   d. Contracted tendon

130. **A single exostosis on a splint bone is known as:**

   a. Simple splint

   b. Chain splint

   c. Knee splint

   d. Peg splint

131. **Several small exostoses in a row on a splint bone are referred to as a:**

   a. Simple splint

   b. Chain splint

   c. Knee splint

   d. Peg splint

132. **An upper third splint which approaches the knee joint is referred as a:**

a. Simple splint

b. Chain splint

c. Knee splint

d. Peg splint

133. **Exostosis on the posterior aspect of a cannon bone between the bone and the suspensory ligament is referred to as a:**

a. Simple splint

b. Chain splint

c. Knee splint

d. Peg splint

134. **A large exostosis on the metacarpal bone is referred to as a:**

a. Jack splint

b. Chain splint

c. Knee splint

d. Peg splint

135. **Uniform thickening of splint bone due to a metabolic disorder is known as a:**

a. Simple splint

b. Spongy splint

c. Knee splint

d. Peg splint

136. **What develops due to a sprain or tear of the interosseous ligament?**

a. True splint

b. Spongy splint

c. Knee splint

d. Peg splint

137. **What develops due to inflammation of the interosseous liga-ment?**

   a. Blind splint

   b. Spongy splint

   c. Knee splint

   d. True splint

138. **Osteoperiostitis involving the cranial aspect of large meta-carpal or large metatarsal bone is known as:**

   a. Sore shin

   b. Buck shin

   c. a and b

   d. None of these

139. **'Sore shin' is also known as:**

   a. Buck shin

   b. Peg splint

   c. Tendonitis

   d. None of these

140. **What is defined as the strain-induced inflammation-involving tendon that is surrounded by paratendon but not the tendon sheath?**

   a. Buck shin

   b. Peg splint

   c. Tendonitis

   d. None of these

141. **Distension of the joint capsule due to synovial effusion is known as:**

   a. Buck shin

   b. Peg splint

   c. Tendonitis

   d. Windpuff

142. **Which of the following conditions does not manifest as lameness?**

    a. Buck shin

    b. Peg splint

    c. Tendonitis

    d. Windpuff

143. **Which of these is defined as the thickening associated with synovitis and capsulitis of the fetlock joint due to trauma?**

    a. Osselets

    b. Ringbone

    c. Quittor

    d. Sidebones

144. **Bony enlargement of the phalanges in the pastern region below the fetlock is called:**

    a. Osselets

    b. Ringbone

    c. Quittor

    d. Sidebones

145. **Which of these is defined as chronic purulent inflammation of a collateral cartilage of the distal phalanx?**

    a. Osselets

    b. Ringbone

    c. Quittor

    d. Sidebones

146. **Ossification of the collateral cartilages of the third phalanx is known as:**

    a. Osselets

    b. Ringbone

    c. Quittor

    d. Sidebones

147. **Which of these is a degenerative disease involving the navicular bone, navicular bursa and deep digital flexor tendon?**

   a. Navicular disease

   b. Ringbone

   c. Quittor

   d. Sidebones

148. **Navicular disease is what in nature?**

   a. Acute

   b. Peracute

   c. Subacute

   d. Chronic

149. **Which of these is characterized by pyramidal distortion of the hoof and distal dorsal pastern region?**

   a. Navicular disease

   b. Ringbone

   c. Buttress foot

   d. Sidebones

150. **Which of these is sometime referred to as the advanced stage of low ringbone?**

   a. Navicular disease

   b. Ringbone

   c. Buttress foot

   d. Sidebones

151. **'Sand crack' is also known as:**

   a. Toe crack

   b. Quarter crack

   c. Heel crack

   d. All of these

152. **Which of these is characterized by the separation of the wall and the sensitive laminae of the foot?**

    a. Seedy toe

    b. Quarter crack

    c. Laminitis

    d. Os pedis

153. **Which of these is a demineralization of the distal phalanx resulting from inflammation?**

    a. Seedy toe

    b. Quarter crack

    c. Pedal osteitis

    d. Os pedis

154. **Upward fixation of the patella is known as:**

    a. Stringhalt

    b. Os pedis

    c. Laminitis

    d. None of these

155. **Stringhalt is hereditary in nature.**

    a. True statement

    b. False statement

    c. a and b

    d. None of these

156. **Which of these is an involuntary flexion of the hock during progression, and may affect one or both hind limbs?**

    a. Stringhalt

    b. Os pedis

    c. Laminitis

    d. None of these

157. **Which digital extensor muscle is involved in the aetiology of string halt?**

   a. Lateral

   b. Medial

   c. Middle

   d. All of these

158. **Tenosynovitis of the tarsal sheath is known as:**

   a. Stringhalt

   b. Os pedis

   c. Laminitis

   d. Thoroughpin

159. **Chronic distension of the tarsocrural joint capsule of the hock, causing swelling of the dorsomedial aspect is known as:**

   a. Bog spavin

   b. Os pedis

   c. Laminitis

   d. Thoroughpin

160. **Enlargement of the plantar aspect of the fibular tarsal bone due to inflammation and thickening of the plantar ligament is referred to as:**

   a. Bog spavin

   b. Curb

   c. Laminitis

   d. Thoroughpin

161. **'Capped hock' is also known as:**

   a. Bog spavin

   b. Curb

   c. Laminitis

   d. Pseudobursitis

162. **The normal pH of synovial fluid is:**

    a. 7.2–7.4

    b. 5.2–5.6

    c. 8.1–8.3

    d. None of these

163. **Osteoblasts are which type of nuclear cells?**

    a. Mono

    b. Multi

    c. Bi

    d. None of these

164. **Which of these refers to inflammation of osseous as well as myeloid bone tissue?**

    a. Osteomyelitis

    b. Osteodystrophy

    c. Infective arthritis

    d. None of these

165. **What is indicated in failure of normal bone development?**

    a. Osteomyelitis

    b. Osteodystrophy

    c. Infective arthritis

    d. None of these

166. **Foot rot is also known as:**

    a. Interdigital necrobacillosis

    b. Interdigital pododermatitis

    c. a and b

    d. None of these

167. **Which of these denotes osteitis resulting from infection?**

    a. Suppurative osteitis

    b. Non-suppurative osteitis

    c. Osteitis deformans

    d. None of these

168. **Which of these diseases affects the vertebrae?**

    a. Ankylosis

    b. Spondylosis

    c. Arthropathy

    d. Dysplasia

169. **Which of these is a disease of the joints?**

    a. Ankylosis

    b. Spondylosis

    c. Arthropathy

    d. Dysplasia

170. **Which of these causes hardening of bony spaces?**

    a. Osteopenia

    b. Osteopetrosis

    c. Epiphysial dysplasia

    d. Osteosclerosis

171. **What type of arthritis would you have if the lining of your joint becomes inflamed?**

    a. Psoriatic arthritis

    b. Osteoarthritis

    c. Rheumatoid arthritis

    d. None of these

172. **Which of these is a chronic disease of the skeleton involving softening of the bone followed by thickening of the cortex?**

    a. Suppurative osteitis

    b. Non-suppurative osteitis

    c. Osteitis deformans

    d. None of these

173. **Coracoid process is absent in which of the following species:**

   a. Dog

   b. Fowl

   c. Ox

   d. Horse

174. **A pulley-like, grooved articular surface is known as what?**

   a. Incisura

   b. Trochlea

   c. Cleft

   d. Condyle

175. **Nutrient foramina is present in which part of the humerus of pigs?**

   a. Distal third of posterior surface

   b. Middle third of posterior surface

   c. a and b

   d. None of these

176. **Teres tubercle give attachment to which of the following muscles:**

   a. Teres major

   b. Latissimus dorsi

   c. a and b

   d. None of these

177. **An atypical cervical vertebra is:**

   a. 1st

   b. 2nd

   c. 6th

   d. 7th

178. **What is the name for the surface of the forelimb that makes contact with the ground when an animal is standing up?**

    a. Interior

    b. Palmar

    c. Plantar

    d. Proximal

179. **What colour are the muscle fibres stained when using H & E stain?**

    a. Blue

    b. Pink

    c. Pinkish-Red

    d. Reddish-Violet

180. **Which bone is part of the axial skeleton?**

    a. Femur

    b. Tibia

    c. Sacrum

    d. Humerus

181. **Which muscle is located in the medial aspect of the thigh region?**

    a. Gluteus medius

    b. Semitendinosus

    c. Biceps femoris

    d. Sartorius

182. **The prepubic tendon is the insertion of _____ muscle.**

    a. Creamaster

    b. Rectus abdominis

    c. Abdominis internus

    d. Transverse abdominis

183. **Which of the following is not a sublumbar muscle?**

    a. Psoas major

    b. Psoas major

    c. Iliacus

    d. Gracilis

184. **What is the total number of bones in an ox?**

    a. 229

    b. 208

    c. 200

    d. 291

185. **The pectoralis is the largest fleshy muscle in which species?**

    a. Oxen

    b. Fowl

    c. Rabbits

    d. Dogs

186. **The medial digital extensor muscle is absent in:**

    a. Horses

    b. Dogs

    c. a and b

    d. None of these

187. **Which of the following is a bone of the arm region?**

    a. Humerus

    b. Radius

    c. Carpal

    d. Metacarpal

188. **The acromin process is absent in:**

    a. Buffalo

    b. Pigs

c. Dogs

d. Donkeys

189. **The 'pin bone' is also known as the:**

a. Ilium

b. Ischium

c. Pubis

d. Sacrum

190. **Fossa ovalis is a depression present at the superior aspect of what?**

a. Posterior venacava

b. Interarterial septum

c. Interventrical septum

d. Atrio-ventricular septum

191. **Perichondrium is absent in which type of cartilage?**

a. Hyaline

b. Elastic

c. Fibro-elastic

d. All of these

192. **The first cervical vertebra is called the:**

a. Atlas

b. Axis

c. a and b

d. None of these

193. **Deltoid tuberosity is present on the anterio-lateral aspect of what?**

a. Radius

b. Ulna

c. Humerus

d. Femur

194. **Select the incorrect one regarding bones involved in given joint of the body:**

    a. Shoulder joint: scapula and humerus

    b. Stifle joint: femur and tibia

    c. Knee joint: tibia, tarsal and metatarsal

    d. Elbow joint: humerus and radius ulna

195. **Select the incorrect one regarding visceral bone present in animals:**

    a. Os penis – dog

    b. Os cordis – pig

    c. Os phrenic – camel

    d. Os opticus – fowl

196. **Which statement is incorrect regarding the humerus:**

    a. Deltoid tuberosity is prominent in cows

    b. Teres tubercle is absent in cows

    c. Supratrochlear foramen is present in the humerus of pigs

    d. Nutrient foramen is present at the medial surface of the humerus in equines

197. **Select the incorrect statement regarding the scapula:**

    a. The acromin process is absent in horses

    b. The coracoid process is absent in pigs

    c. The subscapular fossa is absent in dogs

    d. The glenoid notch is rudimentary in cattle

198. **Upward fixation of the patella is referred to as:**

    a. Stringhalt

    b. Os pedis

    c. Laminitis

    d. None of these

199. **A superficial or deep wound on the knees is called as:**

   a. Paralysis of the radial nerve

   b. Broken knee

   c. Omarthritis

   d. Capped elbow

200. **Osteoarthritis occurs as a result of:**

   a. Deficiency of calcium in young people

   b. Low levels of estrogen in older women

   c. Gradual degeneration of the movable joints, due to wear and tear of the articular cartilage,with the advancing age

   d. High levels of estrogen in older women

Answers

1.	c	31.	c	61.	a	91.	d
2.	b	32.	a	62.	b	92.	b
3.	a	33.	b	63.	c	93.	c
4.	b	34.	b	64.	d	94.	a
5.	a	35.	c	65.	b	95.	b
6.	b	36.	a	66.	a	96.	b
7.	a	37.	d	67.	b	97.	c
8.	a	38.	c	68.	a	98.	a
9.	a	39.	c	69.	b	99.	d
10.	c	40.	a	70.	c	100.	c
11.	c	41.	b	71.	d	101.	c
12.	b	42.	b	72.	d	102.	a
13.	a	43.	c	73.	d	103.	b
14.	b	44.	d	74.	b	104.	c
15.	b	45.	b	75.	c	105.	a
16.	d	46.	a	76.	a	106.	b
17.	a	47.	d	77.	b	107.	c
18.	b	48.	d	78.	a	108.	d
19.	c	49.	c	79.	b	109.	a
20.	a	50.	b	80.	a	110.	b
21.	a	51.	a	81.	c	111.	c
22.	d	52.	b	82.	a	112.	d
23.	a	53.	c	83.	a	113.	a
24.	b	54.	d	84.	b	114.	b
25.	c	55.	c	85.	c	115.	c
26.	b	56.	a	86.	d	116.	d
27.	c	57.	b	87.	a	117.	a
28.	c	58.	c	88.	a	118.	a
29.	c	59.	d	89.	c	119.	c
30.	d	60.	b	90.	b	120.	b

(Continued)

121.	d	**141.**	d	**161.**	d	**181.**	d
122.	b	**142.**	d	**162.**	a	**182.**	b
123.	b	**143.**	a	**163.**	a	**183.**	d
124.	c	**144.**	b	**164.**	a	**184.**	b
125.	a	**145.**	c	**165.**	b	**185.**	b
126.	b	**146.**	d	**166.**	c	**186.**	c
127.	c	**147.**	a	**167.**	a	**187.**	a
128.	b	**148.**	d	**168.**	b	**188.**	d
129.	d	**149.**	c	**169.**	c	**189.**	b
130.	a	**150.**	c	**170.**	d	**190.**	b
131.	b	**151.**	d	**171.**	c	**191.**	c
132.	c	**152.**	a	**172.**	c	**192.**	a
133.	d	**153.**	c	**173.**	a	**193.**	c
134.	a	**154.**	d	**174.**	b	**194.**	c
135.	b	**155.**	b	**175.**	a	**195.**	b
136.	a	**156.**	a	**176.**	c	**196.**	b
137.	a	**157.**	a	**177.**	a	**197.**	b
138.	c	**158.**	d	**178.**	b	**198.**	d
139.	a	**159.**	a	**179.**	d	**199.**	b
140.	c	**160.**	b	**180.**	c	**200.**	c

www.ingramcontent.com/pod-product-compliance
Lightning Source LLC
Chambersburg PA
CBHW051432270326
41935CB00018B/1802